ANATOMY AND PHYSIOLOGY STUDY GUIDE FOR SPEECH AND HEARING

Second Edition

William R. Culbertson, Ph.D.

Stephanie C. Christensen, Ph.D.

Dennis C. Tanner, Ph.D.

Northern Arizona University
Flagstaff, Arizona

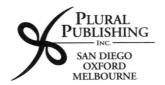

PLURAL
PUBLISHING
INC.

SAN DIEGO
OXFORD
MELBOURNE

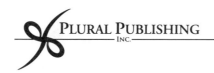

5521 Ruffin Road
San Diego, CA 92123

e-mail: info@pluralpublishing.com
Web site: http://www.pluralpublishing.com

Typeset in 12/14 Helvetica by Flanagan's Publishing Services, Inc.
Printed in the United States of America by McNaughton & Gunn

Library of Congress Cataloging-in-Publication Data is available.
ISBN-13: 978-1-59756-496-0
ISBN-10: 1-59756-496-6

Contents

The *Anatomy and Physiology Guide for Speech and Hearing* is intended to augment a one-semester (or two quarters) undergraduate course in anatomy and physiology of human communication. Students should regard this material as only one of several training modalities in this field.

The authors have upgraded this second edition to include an *Active Learning Guide*. The *Active Learning Guide* contains information to help students respond to items in the workbook. This section contains written material as suggested responses to blank spaces in the Study Outlines as well as simple sketches to fill the empty boxes in the Study Outline units.

The words "anatomy" and "physiology" often intimidate the entry level student. Course titles such as these create thoughts of memorizing long lists of Latin words and trying to comprehend vague concepts of bodily sites and functions. These fears are well founded if the student tries to absorb advanced material from the start. All too often, the result is an elaborate vocabulary built upon a poor foundation, and the student may feel overwhelmed.

The authors intentionally omitted a large amount of information from the content of these units. This was not because the material was unimportant, but because there is only so much material an undergraduate student should be expected to learn and retain at the introductory level. The purpose of this workbook is to help a student develop a starting point from which to search for additional information as the need arises.

There are many fine texts available in anatomy and physiology that contain important material beyond that covered in this workbook. Much or most of it is better advanced to "reference" status. Some additional texts are listed in the reference section.

On top of the need to simplify the material for the student, there is the matter of time. Most communication sciences programs allow one term for anatomy and physiology courses. Professors may find themselves lecturing rapidly, like radio announcers, to include all the material within the time limits of the term. Limitations on the extent of this workbook resulted from many years of full-time clinical and teaching experience.

The units are designed according to a three-step study sequence. First, the student should become familiar with the stated **Goals**, and check these again at the completion of the unit. Accomplishment of the goals should provide a very well-rounded idea of anatomy and physiology as it generally applies to the practice of speech-language pathology and audiology.

Next, the student should follow the **Study Outline**. Study Outlines map the course of study, and are arranged to help students reach unit goals. They list important concepts, structures and/or functions, arranged in progressively smaller "chunks," to ease the assimilation of each topic.

These outlines include italicized questions and activities to help students absorb the material. Space is provided to write the necessary and relevant descriptions, definitions, and/or explanations, but the assiduous student may need additional space in a separate notebook. The information required to complete the outlines may come from many sources, including text(s), a rapidly growing array of online resources, human specimens, models, slides, videos, lectures, and, of course, the *Active Learning Guide*. Instructors may add or delete topics according to course requirements.

Finally, after the student feels comfortable with the material, she or he should take the **Self-Tests**, review the answers, and regard the incorrect ones as feedback on the extent to which the unit is completed. The uses of the self-tests are limited by the student's imagination and personal tastes. A student may use the test as a private means of checking study progress, or use them in groups and share the results. The instructor may employ these tests to allow practice in the class, or for reducing anxiety associated with an actual examination. They provide a valuable learning experience.

The illustrations in this workbook accompany the self-tests. Students should fill in the blanks with the names of the structures indicated. Copies of these illustrations are in the section with the answers to the self-tests. The authors wish to acknowledge the patience and hard work of Susan Durning and Erica Fuchs in the preparation of these illustrations.

A solid background in anatomy and physiology can help the aspiring speech-language pathologist or audiologist prepare for the profession in a stimulating and productive way. The purpose of this workbook is to help establish that background. If the study of anatomy and physiology can become more enjoyable through this workbook, then the authors' hopes will have been realized as well.

PART I

STUDY OUTLINE UNITS

UNIT 1

INTRODUCTION TO ANATOMY AND PHYSIOLOGY

As students begin the study of anatomy and physiology for speech and hearing, they should absorb some general ideas and basic concepts. The ancient study of the forms and functions of the human body is as rooted in culture as it is in science. Terms and concepts about human life vary with language and philosophy.

The anatomical terms used in this workbook are based on the Terminologica Anatomica (TA), conceived in 1998, in Paris, France. TA contains terms in Latin and the equivalent English.

Introduction to anatomy and physiology starts with presentations of the disciplines, including their focuses, similarities and differences. Next, the student should examine specializations within each field to gain appreciation for the breadth of study that is possible.

The introductory section presents guidelines for learning the language of anatomy and physiology in the speech and hearing sciences. Terms apply to **structures** and **locations**, **positions** and **relationships**, and **processes** and **actions**. Mastery of the information contained in the first unit will provide a solid foundation for mastery of material in future units.

The following are the objectives for the unit on the introduction to anatomy and physiology. Success in accomplishing these objectives should prepare the student for further study of the following units. The student may check the appropriate box as each goal is completed in reflection of his or her mastery of the material.

1. Differentiate between the sciences of anatomy and physiology.

2. Describe the following subdivisions of anatomy:
   a. descriptive or systemic anatomy
   b. applied or practical anatomy
   c. microscopic anatomy
   d. developmental anatomy
   e. geriatric anatomy

3. Describe the following subdivisions of physiology:
   a. general physiology
   b. applied physiology
   c. experimental physiology
   d. special physiology
   e. pathologic physiology

4. Describe anatomical position with reference to:
   a. the posture of the body
   b. the position of the limbs
   c. the direction of the eyes
   d. the position of the palms

5. Given diagrams of the human form from different perspectives, identify the following planes:
   a. median or midsagittal plane
   b. sagittal plane
   c. coronal plane
   d. transverse or horizontal plane

✐ ☐   6.   After defining the following anatomical terms, use them to describe the location of any structure or to compare the locations of two or more structures:

   a.   peripheral/central
   b.   ventral/dorsal
   c.   anterior/posterior
   d.   superficial/deep
   e.   superior/inferior
   f.   medial/lateral
   g.   proximal/distal
   h.   caudal/rostral (cranial)
   i.   external/internal

I.   **Definitions**

Fill in the spaces below with the definitions of each science. How do the sciences of anatomy and physiology complement one another?

A.   Anatomy

B.   Physiology

II. **Subdivisions of Anatomy**

Describe each of the following specialized branches in the science of anatomy. Which branches have the most direct relevance to speech-language pathology and audiology? Explain the relevance.

A.   Descriptive Anatomy

B.   Applied Anatomy

C.   Microscopic Anatomy

D.   Developmental Anatomy

E.   Geriatric Anatomy

III.   Subdivisions of Physiology

Fill in the spaces with your definitions of the following specialized branches of physiology. Describe how each has relevance to the fields of audiology and speech-language pathology.

A.   General Physiology

B.   Applied Physiology

C.   Experimental Physiology

D.   Special Physiology

E.   Pathologic Physiology

IV.   Anatomical Position

Why is it important to have a conventional anatomical position?

A.   Position

In the box provided, draw a figure of a person in the anatomical position using the following guidelines:

1.   Body standing erect

2.   Face forward

3.   Arms extended downward at sides

4.   Palms forward

B.   Names of Major Topographical Regions

Locate the following regions in your drawing:

1.   Cranial Region
2.   Cervical Region
3.   Thoracic Region
4.   Abdominal Region
5.   Upper Extremities
6.   Lower Extremities

V.   Anatomical Planes of Reference

Into which sections do these planes divide the body?

A.   Sagittal

B.   Coronal

C.   Transverse (Horizontal)

VI.   Anatomical Location Terms Presented as Antonyms (Opposites)

In which directions do these terms direct the student? Use each term in a sentence to describe the relationship between two familiar body parts.

Peripheral	Central

Ventral	Dorsal

Anterior	Posterior

Superficial	Deep

Superior	Inferior

Medial	Lateral

Proximal	Distal

Caudal	Rostral (Cranial)

External	Internal

1. The human form, in the anatomical position, is situated with the body posture _____, the palms _____, the face _____, and the upper extremities _____.

2. The science that studies the functions of living organisms or their parts is _____.

3. The body is divided into anterior and posterior sections by a _____ plane.

4. The body is divided into superior and inferior sections by a _____ plane.

5. The head is _____ to the shoulder.

6. The heel is _____ to the knee.

7. The brain lies inside the skull. The nose is _____ to the brain.

8. The ear lies on the _____ aspect of the skull.

9. The hand is _____ to the elbow.

10. The science that is concerned with the structure of organisms is called _____.

11. The branch of anatomy that deals with the form of the long-lived individual is called _____.

12. The branch of anatomy that deals with the growth of the organism from a single cell to birth is _____ anatomy.

13. The branch of physiology that deals with the changes brought about by the process of disease is _____ physiology.

14.   Research in speech/language pathology is primarily studied in _____ physiology.

UNIT 2

CYTOLOGY AND HISTOLOGY

Familiarity with the basic components of a system provides a foundation for understanding the larger structure and the scope of its functions. For the biological mechanisms of human communication, the study of cells and tissues is a good place to start.

Elements comprise molecules that, in myriad aggregations, make up the various proteins. Proteins form the components of cells, and serve the cells' essential functions through their chemical reactions. At some point, the basic elemental substrates become **alive**.

The attributes that define life invite the deepest contemplation. Living cells aggregate to form the various **tissues** of which our **organs** are formed. Organs interact and coordinate through **systems** to maintain the complex organism.

The single cell represents the unit constituent of the living body. The human body's genetic code causes proliferation and differentiation of the **zygote**, begun as a single cell product of **gamete** union.

Three basic germ layers appear and become the source for the **four basic tissue types**: **epithelial**, **connective**, **muscle**, and **nervous**. Each type has special properties.

As the **zygote** develops into an **embryo**, and nine weeks after fertilization, into a **fetus**, discrete structures become visible. Early in fetal development, small arch-shaped ripples appear in its rostral end. These arches are called **branchial arches**. They form the foundations of most of the structures we associate with the peripheral speech and hearing mechanisms.

The human communication mechanism is efficient at its task partly because it is composed of specialized tissues. Special types of connective and epithelial tissues respond to the vibrations of sound energy and air compression to transmit and receive the signals we call speech. Muscle tissue, by virtue of its contractibility, and nervous tissue, through its enhanced excitability, allows the individual to make sounds with the gases of respiration.

Most books on anatomy and physiology consider the body as divided into convenient sections. This division eases study, but the advanced student will soon learn to appreciate the synergy with which all systems must operate. All **cells**, **tissues**, **organs**, and **systems** interact to form a unity in the healthy individual.

The following are the goals for the unit on basic human cells and tissues. The student can determine mastery of the material presented in this unit by checking the appropriate box as each goal as completed.

✎ ☐   1.   Define and give examples of each of these structural units:
a.   cell
b.   tissue
c.   organ
d.   system

✎ ☐   2.   List the qualities that describe the property of life.

✎ ☐   3.   Describe the cell in terms of its basic substance and two principal constituents.

✎ ☐   4.   Name and describe the four basic tissue types of the human body.

✎ ☐   5.   Name and describe the three functional and three anatomical names for articulations (classifications of joints).

✎ ☐   6.   Describe the three germ layers of the developing embryo and major tissues that derive from each.

✎ ☐   7.   Describe branchial arches and the general functions of their derivative structures.

I.   **General Notes**

Fill in the spaces below with the definitions.

A.   **Cytology**

B.   **Histology**

II.   **Cytology**

Fill in the cytological definitions in the spaces provided.

A.   **Cell**

B.   **Characteristics of Living Matter**

1.   **Characteristics of Life in *All* Organisms**

In your own words, describe the following characteristics that distinguish living matter from that which is not living.

a.   **Growth**

b.   **Reproduction**

c.   **Metabolism**

d.   Adaptation or Irritability

2.   Characteristics of Life in *Some* Organisms

Define the following characteristics. Under each category provide an example of a living organism that does not exhibit the characteristic.

a.   Spontaneous Movement

b.   Expression of Consciousness

c.   Voluntary Use of Senses

C.   General Structure of the Cell

Briefly describe the parts and functions of these fundamental cell components.

1.   Protoplasm

2.   Cytoplasm

3.   Nucleus

4.   Cell Fluids

5.   **Cell Shape**

What are some common cell shapes?
In the boxes provided, draw cells of three different shapes.

III.   **Histology**

Fill in the fundamental histological definitions in the spaces provided.

A.   **Definition of Tissue**

B.   **Four Basic Tissue Types**

Describe the form and function of the following tissue types. Provide at least one specific example of a structure in the human speech and hearing mechanism made up of each tissue type.

1.   **Epithelial**

2.   **Connective**

3.   **Muscle**

4.   **Nervous**

C. Epithelial Tissue

1. Characteristics of Epithelial Tissue

Describe the following aspects of epithelial tissue in the spaces provided.

a. Intercellular Structure

b. Cellular Arrangement

2. Functions of Epithelial Tissue

Explain how epithelial tissue performs the following functions.

a. Protective

b. Absorptive

c. Secretory

d. Glandular

e. Sensory

3.   Types of Epithelial Tissue

Describe the following types of epithelial tissues. Where might they be found within the mechanism for communication?

a.   Proper Epithelium

b.   Mesothelium

c.   Endothelium

4.   Descriptive Terms of Epithelial Tissue

Define these terms that classify epithelial tissue.

a.   Cell Shape

In the boxes provided, draw pictures of the following cell shapes.

(1)   Squamous   (3)   Pyramidal

(2)   Columnar   (4)   Cuboidal

b. Layers

(1) Simple

(2) Stratified

D. Connective Tissue

1. Characteristics of Connective Tissue

In the spaces below, describe the following aspects of connective tissue.

a. Variability of Intercellular Structure

b. Variability of Form

2. Functions of Connective Tissue

Explain how connective tissue performs the following functions.

a. Structural Binding

b. Structural Separation

c. Fatty Connective Tissue Functions

d.   Fluid Connective Tissue Functions

3.   Types of Connective Tissue

Describe each type of connective tissue. Give examples of each in the human communication mechanism.

a.   Loose Connective Tissue

(1)   Areolar Tissue

(2)   Adipose Tissue

(3)   Reticular Tissue

b.   Dense Connective Tissue

(1)   Tendons

(2)   Ligaments

(3)   Aponeuroses

(4) Fascia

c. **Skeletal Connective Tissue**

(1) Cartilage

(a) Hyaline

(b) Elastic

(c) Fibrous

(2) Bone

Describe bone in terms of the special nature of its intercellular material. Describe the following types of bones and provide an example of a body structure composed of each bone type.

(a) Long Bone

(b) Short Bone

(c)   Flat Bone

(d)   Irregular Bone

(3)   **Articulations of the Skeletal System**

What does the term "articulation" mean in anatomy and physiology?

(a)   **Functional Classification of Joints**

Describe the direction and extent of movement each joint allows. What are the advantages of each type? Give examples of each type of joint in the human communication mechanism.

i)   Synarthrodial

ii)   Amphiarthrodial

iii)   Diarthrodial

(b)   **Anatomical Classification of Joints**

Describe the following anatomical joint types. To what functional classification does each correspond?

i)   Fibrous

ii)   Cartilaginous

iii)   Synovial

(4)   **Divisions of the Skeletal System**

List the structures that comprise these skeletal divisions.

(a)   **Axial Skeleton**

(b)   **Appendicular Skeleton**

4.   **Fluid Connective Tissue**

What characteristic of the intercellular structure of fluid connective tissue distinguishes it? What are the functions of the two fluid tissues?

a.   **Blood**

b.   **Lymph**

E.   Muscle Tissue

    1.   Characteristics of Muscle Tissue

    Describe the identifying characteristics of muscle tissue.

    2.   Functions of Muscle Tissue

    Describe how muscle tissue functions at these progressively larger contractile units.

        a.   Sarcomere

        b.   Myofibril

        c.   Muscle Fiber

        d.   Muscle Fasciculus

        e.   Muscle

    3.   Types of Muscle Tissue

    Differentiate between the following types of muscle tissue. Where is each type of muscle tissue found?

        a.   Smooth

b.   Cardiac

c.   Striated

4.   Muscle Feedback

What is the role of conscious and unconscious muscle feedback in the regulation of muscle function for speech?

5.   Muscle Attachment

To which end of a muscle do the following terms refer?

a.   Origin

b.   Insertion

6.   Muscle Function Terminology

Define the following muscle function terms and demonstrate your understanding by describing the movement of a body part or body parts in respect to the terms.

a.   Flexion

b.   Extension

      c.   Adduction

      d.   Abduction

7.   **Names of Muscles**

Give examples of muscles named according to the characteristics below.

      a.   Shape

      b.   Function

      c.   Location

F.   **Nervous Tissue**

1.   **Characteristics of Nervous Tissue**

Describe the following special aspects of nervous tissue.

      a.   Excitability

      b.   Conductivity

2.   **Functions of Nervous Tissue**

Explain how nervous tissue performs the following functions.

   a.   **Excitatory**

   b.   **Inhibitory**

3.   **Types of Nervous Tissue**

   a.   **Neurons**

   Describe the following types of neurons. Give examples of locations at which each may be found in the mechanism for human communication.

   (1)   **Unipolar Neurons**

   (2)   **Bipolar Neurons**

   (3)   **Multipolar Neurons**

In the boxes provided, draw stylized representations of each type and label the cell body, axons, and dendrites.

b.   **Neuroglial Cells**

Describe the following neuroglial cells. What are their unique functions?

(1)   **Myelinating Glia**

(2)   **Astrocytes**

(3)   **Microglia**

(4)   **Neurilemma (Ependymal Cells)**

G. Tissue Differentiation

1. Germ Layers

Define each of the following germ layers in the spaces provided. Give examples of organs or structures in the speech or hearing mechanism derived from each.

a. Endoderm

b. Mesoderm

c. Ectoderm

2. Branchial Arches

What is a branchial arch? At which end of the embryo do they appear?

List the speech and hearing structures that develop from each arch in the spaces provided.

a. First Arch (Mandibular Arch)

b. Second Arch (Hyoid Arch)

c. Third Arch

        d.   Fourth Arch

        e.   Fifth Arch

        f.   Sixth Arch

III.   Organs and Systems

    A.   Definitions

        Fill in the following definitions in the spaces provided.

        1.   System

        2.   Organ

    B.   Review of Systems and Their Interactions

        What are the life-sustaining functions of the following systems? Which ones have overlaid communicative functions?

        1.   Respiratory

        2.   Nervous

        3.   Muscular

4. Circulatory

5. Digestive

6. Urinary

7. Endocrine

8. Vascular

9. Skeletal

10. Integumentary

11. Articular

1. A cell is composed of _____.

2. Four characteristics that identify an entity as being alive are:

   a. _____

   b. _____

   c. _____

   d. _____

3. The study of collections of cells that have similar structures and functions is called _____.

4. The thicker part of the protoplasm of a cell is called the _____.

5. Name the tissue types that have the following special characteristics:

   a. Characterized by irritability. _____

   b. Forms a protective sheath covering the interior and exterior surfaces of the body. _____

   c. Mediates body movements by virtue of contractile properties. _____

   d. Binds the body structures together and aids in body maintenance. _____

   e. Conducts changes in electrical potential. _____

6. Indicate from which germ layers the following structures are derived:

   a. The brain _____

   b. The muscles of the tongue _____

   c. The cranial nerves _____

   d. The jaw bone _____

e. The lungs _____

7. The branchial skeleton includes the _____ and _____ bones, as well as the _____ and _____ cartilages.

8. The primary function of the branchial and hypobranchial musculature is _____.

9. Embryonic cells differentiate into three distinct groups called _____.

10. Joints that move freely are called _____ or _____.

11. The type of muscle that is under voluntary control is _____.

12. What comprises a *motor unit*? _____

13. The term applied to the attachment of a muscle to a more movable body part is _____.

14. Define *organ*.

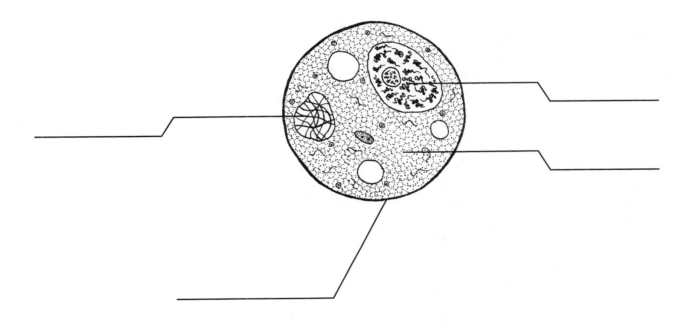

SOMATIC CELL

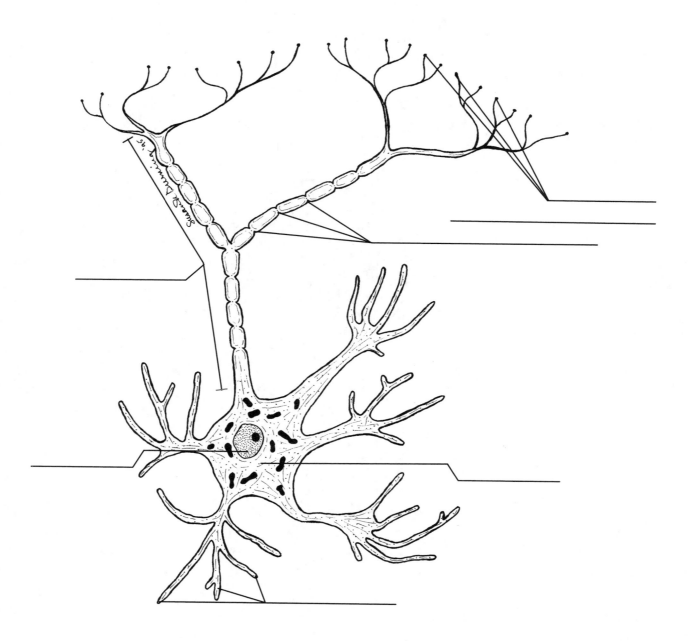

NEURON

UNIT 3

THE RESPIRATORY MECHANISM

The essential function of the respiratory system is to allow the exchange of gasses to and from the environment. By virtue of its specialized structure, the respiratory mechanism allows the exchange of **oxygen** from the external atmosphere for **carbon dioxide** from the bloodstream. While the life function of respiration is automatic, human beings have learned to control the respiratory system for the overlaid function of speaking.

The phase in which air flows into the lungs is referred to as **inspiration**. Air, and other liquids and gases, flow from higher pressure regions to lower pressure regions. An inward flow of oxygen containing atmospheric air results from contraction of the muscles of inspiration. More than a dozen muscles are involved in this process. Contractions of these muscles increase the size of the thorax vertically, anteroposteriorly, and transversely. As the size of the thorax increases, the pressure inside decreases according to **Boyle's law**. Certain forces that oppose inspiration must be overcome. They include the small resistance to airflow in the respiratory airway, the resistance to deformation of the respiratory tissue or the elastic recoil of the lungs and thorax, and the fluid pressure of the abdomen.

Expiration is the phase in which air flows from the lungs. This flow is caused by a decrease in the dimensions of the thorax and a resulting increase in its internal pressure. Expiratory changes are normally effected by allowing the forces that oppose inspiration to act. At the peak of inspiration, the alveolar pressure is equal to the atmospheric pressure. When the muscles of inspiration relax, the alveolar pressure exceeds that of the atmosphere and causes air to flow out of the lungs. When forceful expulsion of respiratory air is required, the muscles of expiration contract.

The anatomy of the healthy respiratory mechanism creates a dynamic balance among the structures of the torso. The torso, or the body without the extremities, is divided into superior and inferior divisions by the dome-shaped **diaphragm**. The diaphragm is also the primary muscle of inspiration. The superior division of the torso, containing the heart, lungs, ribs, and muscles, is called the **thorax**. The inferior division is the **abdomen**. This fluid-filled cavity contains the digestive system and various organs and glands. Function of the muscles of respiration alternately shifts the balance of internal and external pressures between and among the thoracic cavities and the external atmosphere.

Viewing the respiratory system as a **biological pump** is a convenient analogy. This pump compresses the air used for vital functions and for speech purposes. Physiological terms for respiratory pressures include **alveolar pressure** or pressure within the lungs and **pleural pressure** or pressure within the thorax but outside the lungs. **Abdominal pressure** is the pressure in the abdomen.

The volumes or air involved in respiratory functions are measured with a spirometer. **Tidal capacity** is the total volume of air expired during each normal respiratory cycle. **Complemental air** is the maximum volume of air that can be inspired beyond normal inspiration and is also known as inspiratory reserve. **Supplemental air**, or expiratory reserve volume, is the maximum volume of air that can be expired beyond the end of a normal tidal expiration. **Residual air** volume is the air remaining in the lungs that cannot be exhaled. **Vital capacity** is the total volume of air measurable within the lungs and includes the sum of tidal capacity, complemental air, and supplemental air. Respiratory rates vary with age and activity. Sleep may decrease the rate by as much as 25%.

Respiration for speech is normally a voluntary act, while vegetative breathing is an autonomic function. For speaking, the muscles of the thorax decrease the air pressure inside the lungs at a rate much quicker than that for quiet breathing. This results in a quick inspiration. Then the muscles slowly relax, so the gas inside the lungs will last longer. The speech segment will be longer.

The pressurized gas from the lungs flows upward to power the larynx and create the other sound sources for speech. Without the power provided by the respiratory system, speech would be a series of oral gestures, accompanied by very little sound.

The respiratory pump provides a driving force for the generation of voiced and unvoiced sounds. It provides the energy necessary for a series of valving events that result in the acoustic characteristics of phonemes. Voluntary respiratory behavior plays an important role in the suprasegmental aspects of speech, including loudness, pitch, emphasis, and pauses.

Successful accomplishment of these objectives should give the student a basic understanding of respiratory function in speech production. Accomplishment of these objectives provides the foundation necessary for application to the evaluation and treatment of speech disorders. When the objective is accomplished, the student may check the box beside each objective.

✎ ☐   1.   Describe two definitions of respiration.

✎ ☐   2.   Describe the mechanics of physical respiration in terms of the principles of Boyle's law.

✎ ☐   3.   List the structures and divisions of the upper and lower respiratory tracts.

✎ ☐   4.   Describe the skeleton of the thorax and abdomen.

✎ ☐   5.   Describe the mechanics and purposes of respiration for life and for speech.

✎ ☐   6.   Describe the muscles of inspiration and their functions.

✎ ☐   7.   Differentiate between the muscles of inspiration and the muscles of expiration.

✎ ☐   8.   Describe the following respiratory volumes:
   a.   Tidal Volume
   b.   Vital Capacity
   c.   Inspiratory Reserve
   d.   Expiratory Reserve
   e.   Residual Volume

✎ ☐   9.   Describe the different respiratory patterns, including:
   a.   Diaphragmatic/Abdominal
   b.   Thoracic
   c.   Clavicular
   d.   Cheyne-Stokes
   e.   Neurogenic Hyperventilation
   f.   Kussmaul Respiration

✎ ☐   10.   Describe chronic diseases of the respiratory tract, including asthma, emphysema, chronic bronchitis, and chronic obstructive pulmonary disease (COPD).

I. Two Definitions for Respiration

What are the two primary functions of the respiratory system and why is respiration important to speech-language pathologists? Fill in the definitions in the spaces provided.

    A.   Physical Respiration

        1.   Biological Functions

        2.   Speech Function

    B.   Chemical Respiration

Include the chemical equation for respiration.

II. Structures of the Respiratory Tract

    A.   Location of the Respiratory System

Describe the general location of the structures for breathing. Which ones are located in the upper part?

        1.   Upper Respiratory Tract

        2.   Lower Respiratory Tract

B.   Skeleton of the Respiratory Tract

Describe the location of the following structures and indicate how many of each are in the body.

1.   Spinal Column

a.   Vertebrae

(1)   Structure

Describe the general structure of a vertebra.

(2)   Types of Vertebrae

To which vertebrae do these names refer? How many of each are there?

(a)   Cervical

i)   Special Names for Cervical Vertebrae

Describe the location of each of these vertebrae.

a)   Atlas

b)   Axis

c)   Vertebra Prominens

(b)   Thoracic

(c)   Lumbar

(d)   Sacral

(e)   Coccygeal

2.   **Pelvic Girdle**

What is the role of the pelvic girdle in respiration?

3.   **Rib Cage**

a.   **Ribs**

b.   **Sternum**

4.   **Clavicles**

5. Scapulae

C. Nose and Nasal Cavity

1. Nares

2. Septum

3. Root

4. Choanae

D. Pharynx

Differentiate between these subdivisions of the pharynx.

1. Nasopharynx

2. Oropharynx

3. Laryngopharynx

E. **Oral Cavity Structure and Function**

   Describe the locations of these oral landmarks.

   1. **Fauces**

   2. **Triangular Fossa**

   3. **Tonsils**

F. **Laryngopharynx**

   What is the respiratory function of the larynx?

G. **Trachea**

   Describe the structure and location of the trachea. What is its location relative to the esophagus?

H. **Bronchial Tree**

   Differentiate between the following components of the bronchial tree by their location in relation to one another.

   1. **Main Stem Bronchi**

   2. **Secondary Bronchi**

3.   Tertiary Bronchi

4.   Bronchioles

I.   Lungs

Describe the following structures and characteristics of the lungs in the spaces provided.

1.   Right and Left Lung Differences

2.   Alveoli

3.   Pleurae

a.   Intrapleural Fluid

b.   Visceral Pleura

c.   Parietal Pleura

III.   **Mechanics of Respiration**

How does Boyle's law relate to breathing? Demonstrate your understanding by providing an example of Boyle's law at work in something other than respiration.

A.   **Boyle's Law**

B.   **Inspiration and Expiration**

1.   **Respiratory Cycle**

Define a respiratory cycle. What is the normal I-Fraction (ratio of the duration of inspiration to the duration of the entire cycle) for quiet breathing? Describe the differences between the respiratory cycle for speech and that for quiet breathing.

a.   **Vegetative Breathing**

b.   **Respiration for Speech**

2.   **Respiratory Rates**

What is respiratory rate and how is it measured? What are normal rates for an adult, child, and infant?

a.   **Adult Respiratory Rate Range**

b.   **Child Respiratory Rate Range**

c.   **Infant Respiratory Rate Range**

3. **Respiratory Patterns**

   Describe the most commonly encountered patterns of respiration? How does the diagnostician identify one? Is there one pattern that is more efficient?

   a. **Normal Patterns of Respiration**

      (1) **Diaphragmatic/Abdominal**

      (2) **Thoracic**

      (3) **Clavicular**

   b. **Pathological Patterns of Respiration**

      Describe these pathological patterns of respiration.

      (1) **Cheyne-Stokes Respiration**

      (2) **Neurogenic Hyperventilation**

      (3) **Kussmaul Respiration**

C.   Muscles of Respiration

    1.   Function of the Muscles of Respiration

        How do the following movements bring about changes in thoracic volumes?

        a.   Diaphragmatic Movement

        b.   Costal Movement

            (1)   Pump Handle

            (2)   Bucket Handle

    2.   Inspiration: Active Movement

        a.   Primary Muscles of Inspiration

        Describe the origins and insertions of these muscles.

            (1)   Diaphragm

            (2)   External Intercostals

b.   Secondary Muscles of Inspiration

Under what conditions will an individual employ these muscles? Describe their origins and insertions.

(1)   Pectoralis Majorus/Minoris

(2)   Costal Levators

    (a)   12 paired

    (b)   C-7 to T-11

(3)   Serratus Anteriorus

(4)   Serratus Posterior Superiorus

(5)   Latissimus Dorsi

(6)   Scalenus

    (a)   C-3 through C-6

    (b)   To Ribs 1 and 2

3.   **Expiration**

Describe the different manners in which gas is expelled from the respiratory system.

a.   **Passive Movement**

b.   **Active Movement**

(1)   **Muscles of Expiration**

What is the role of the muscles of expiration in the production of speech?

(a)   **Primary Muscles of Expiration**

Describe the origins and insertions of these muscles.

i)   **Internal Intercostals**

ii)   **Rectus Abdominus**

iii)   **Transversus Abdominus**

iv)   **External Obliques**

v)   **Internal Obliques**

(b)   **Secondary Muscles of Expiration**

Describe the origins and insertions of the secondary muscles of expiration. Under what circumstances might they be employed?

i)   **Serratus Posterior Inferiorus**

ii)   **Quadratus Lumborum**

iii)   **Subcostals**

iv)   **Latissimus Dorsi**

IV.   **Measurement of Respiratory Function**

What are the implications of respiratory function testing in the evaluation and treatment of communicative disorders?

A.   **Spirometry**

Describe the spirometer. Can a speech-language pathologist estimate respiratory efficiency for speech without instrumentation? If so, how?

B.   **Volumes**

Define the following respiratory volumes. What are normal values?

1.   **Vital Capacity**

2.   Tidal

3.   Inspiratory Reserve (Complimentary)

4.   Expiratory Reserve (Supplementary)

5.   Residual

V.   Diseases of the Respiratory System

Describe these common chronic diseases of respiration. What limitations might be imposed of the effects of speech therapy for individuals suffering from these conditions?

A.   Asthma

B.   Chronic Obstructive Pulmonary Disease (COPD)

1.   Emphysema

2.   Chronic Bronchitis

1. What are the two points of view from which we can describe respiration?

   _____ and _____.

2. Air moves in and out of the respiratory tract coincident with changes in the

   _____ of the thorax in a manner consistent with which law of physics?

   _____

3. Identify the following anatomical structures as belonging to either the *upper* or *lower* respiratory tract.

   a. Nasopharynx _____   f. Bronchi _____

   b. Lungs _____   g. Pleurae _____

   c. Oral Cavity _____   h. Nostrils _____

   d. Fauces _____   I. Trachea _____

   e. Choanae _____   j. Oropharynx _____

4. The *nonbiological* function of respiration is _____.

5. The respiratory system consists of _____.

6. A respiratory cycle consists of _____.

7. The normal respiratory rate for adults is _____.

8. The operation of Boyle's law is ensured by action of _____.

9. The primary muscles of inspiration are _____.

10. During normal expiration, the muscles of respiration _____.

11. The first seven vertebrae are called _____.

12. The lateral movement of ribs 7 to 10 is referred to as _____.

13. The muscles of expiration contract for _____

    _____.

14. The true ribs attach anteriorly to the _____.

15. A device that measures respiratory volumes is called a _____.

16. The vertebrae closest to the lungs are called _____.

17. The volume of air inhaled and exhaled during any single expiratory cycle is

    called the _____.

18. The quantity of air that can be exhaled after as deep an inspiration as possible

    is called _____.

19. The I-fraction for speech is approximately _____.

20. Expiratory reserve is also known as _____, and is the term used to

    describe the volume of air that _____.

21. The two *normal* patterns of respiration are called _____ and

    _____.

22. Describe Cheyne-Stokes respiration.

23. What are the rehabilitation implications of COPD?

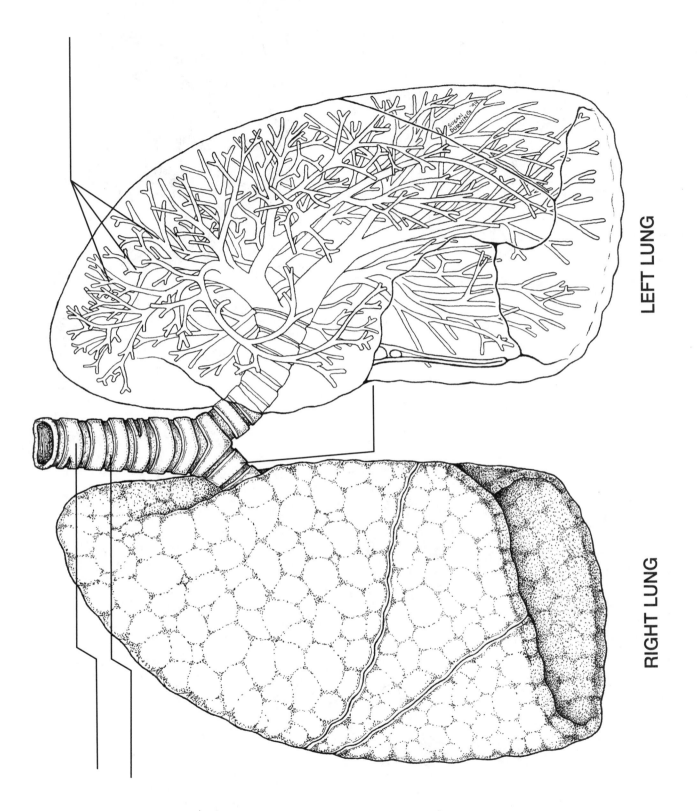

65

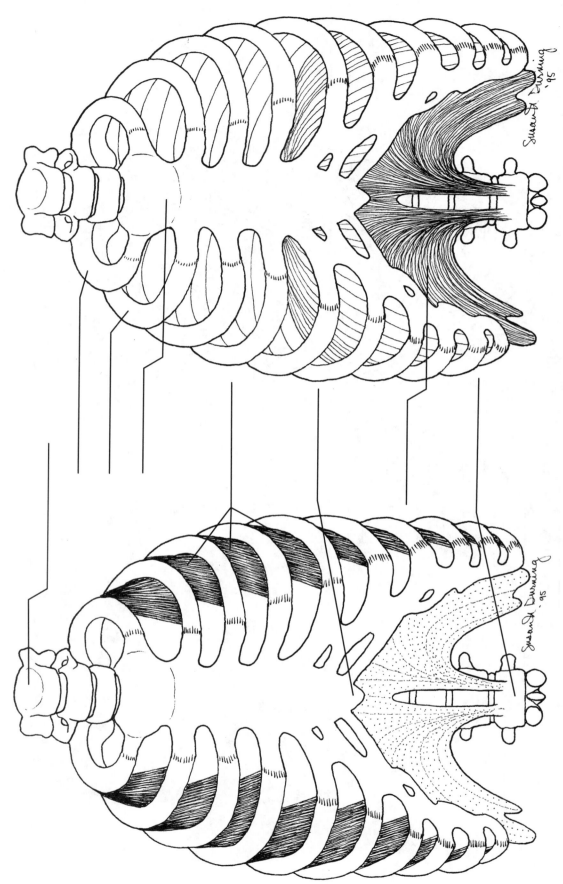

THORACIC SKELETON

UNIT 4

THE PHONATORY MECHANISM

The production of speech depends on the transmission of sound waves. One of the main anatomical locations for sound production is the **larynx**. The larynx functions as a series of three valves. The most inferior of these valves is formed by the vocal folds. Because both food traveling to the stomach and air passing to the lungs begin in the same passage, the larynx serves a dual purpose. It permits the passage of air to and from the lungs while being capable of closing during swallowing to protect the lungs from food and other foreign bodies. The opening at the level of the vocal folds is called the **glottis**. Other functions of the larynx include stabilization of the thorax for body exertions and regulation of airflow in and out of the lungs. **Phonation** refers to any type of vibratory sound produced at the level of the larynx. Whisper is also a function of partially contracting the vocal folds.

The larynx consists of 11 **cartilages** of which four are paired. The largest is the **thyroid cartilage**. The **cricoid cartilage** resembles a signet ring. The **epiglottis**, which is not vital to humans, snaps down like a trap to help protect the airways. The **arytenoid, corniculate, cuneiform,** and **triticeal** cartilages are the paired cartilages.

The cartilages of the larynx are tied to one another by **intrinsic ligaments**. **Extrinsic ligaments** connect the laryngeal cartilages to the hyoid bone, above, and to the first tracheal ring, below. In addition to their functions as connecting tissues, the intrinsic laryngeal ligaments, spread thin in some places to form membranes, play roles in producing the vibrations we associate with the voice.

The musculature of the phonatory mechanism moves its structure to adjust its openings and postures. **Intrinsic laryngeal muscles** have both origins and insertions within the laryngeal structure. They are essential to pitch and loudness control. Only one muscle is responsible for opening, or abducting, the vocal folds: the posterior crico-arytenoid. Adductors are intrinsic muscles responsible for forcefully closing the vocal folds. Tensors and relaxers work to elongate and shorten the vocal folds. **Extrinsic laryngeal muscles** have one or more connections outside the larynx and are frequently referred to as either suprahyoid or infrahyoid. Suprahyoid muscles help elevate the larynx whereas infrahyoids (neck strap muscles) are involved in lowering it.

The larynx comprises a portion of the pharynx. This portion is called the **laryngo-pharynx.** It is divided into three cavities. At the superior end in the vestibular portion. This is the entrance to the airway. The middle division of the laryngopharynx is the ventricle. It is bordered by two sets of tissue folds: the **ventricular (false) vocal folds** at the superior end and the **(true) vocal folds** at the inferior end. Inferior to the ventricle is the **subglottal area** of the laryngopharynx.

The act of producing voiced speech is dependent on respiratory support. The vocal folds rapidly vibrate as the compressed respiratory air travels over their surfaces. The vocal folds are capable of closing rapidly due to both **myoelastic** properties of the laryngeal tissue and the **aerodynamic** Bernoulli principle.

Pitch modulation of glottal wave frequency and glottal wave amplitude result from fine regulation and coordination between subglottal air pressure and muscle resistance. During elevation of pitch, the mass per unit length of the vocal folds is decreased. Lowering of the pitch is a result of an increase of mass per unit length of the vocal folds. To effect these mass changes, the vocalis muscle and the vocal ligament are adjusted by fine movements of the arytenoid cartilages which are capable of sliding and rotating in response to intrinsic muscle tension and length. Modulation of glottal wave amplitude results from variations in subglottal air pressure, counterbalanced by variations in vocal fold muscular resistance.

Mastery of the following objectives will give the student a basic understanding of the form and function of the mechanism used to produce the voice. Such an understanding will give the student a point of departure for study of the evaluation and treatment of phonatory disorders. Students should check the boxes by the objectives as they accomplish them.

1. Describe the larynx in terms of its physical appearance, location, and functions.

2. Describe the general process of phonation and the glottic cycle.

3. Describe glottal postures and their effects on phonatory source characteristics.

4. Name and identify the major cartilages of the larynx.

5. Describe the articulations of the major laryngeal cartilages.

6. Name and identify the major ligaments and membranes of the larynx.

7. Name and identify the intrinsic muscles of the larynx.

8. Name and identify the three sections of the cavity of the larynx.

9. Differentiate the functions of the intrinsic versus the extrinsic muscles of the larynx.

I.   General Structure and Function

    A.   General Description and Location

        Describe the larynx and its general location.

    B.   Evolution

        What is the function of the larynx in lower animals?

    C.   Biological Function

        Apart from phonation, what are the functions of the laryngeal valve?

    D.   Speech Function

        What is the speech function of the larynx? How does it accomplish this function?

1. **The Glottis and Vocal Folds**

   What is the glottis? Differentiate between abduction and adduction of the vocal folds.

   a. **Abduction**

   b. **Adduction**

2. **Physiology of Normal Phonation**

   a. **The Glottal Cycle**

      Describe the following phases of the glottal cycle. Draw a graph of the glottal cycle including percentages of time in each phase to demonstrate your understanding.

      (1) **Closed Phase**

      (2) **Open Phase**

          (a) **Opening Phase**

          (b) **Closing Phase**

(3)   **Forces**

Describe the forces at work during the glottal cycle.

(a)   **Myoelastic**

(b)   **Aerodynamic**

b.   **Glottal Frequency**

What are the effects of changes in glottal frequency?

(1)   **Average Glottal Frequency**

(a)   **Males**

(b)   **Females**

(2)   **Mechanism for Changing Glottal Frequency**

How do the vocal folds change as pitch increases? How are these changes brought about (i.e., what muscles are responsible for altering pitch)?

c.   **Glottal Cycle Amplitude**

Describe changes that occur in the glottal cycle as the voice becomes louder.

II.   The Framework of the Larynx

   A.   The Hyoid Bone

   Is the hyoid bone part of the larynx?

      1.   Structure

         a.   Corpus

         b.   Greater Cornua

         c.   Lesser Cornua

      2.   Function of the Hyoid Bone

         a.   Attachments

         b.   Relationship to Tongue and to Larynx

   B.   Cartilages of the Larynx

   What types of cartilages form the skeleton of the larynx?

1.   **Unpaired Cartilages of the Larynx**

a.   **Thyroid Cartilage**

Describe the Thyroid Cartilage. What is its size relative to the other laryngeal cartilages?

(1)   **Structure**

(a)   **Laminae**

Describe the angle of fusion of the thyroid laminae. How does this angle change as the individual develops? Is there any relationship between this angle and the sound of the voice?

(b)   **Cornua**

b.   **Cricoid Cartilage**

(1)   **Attachments**

What are the superior and inferior attachments of the cricoid cartilage?

(2)   **Structure**

Describe and be able to identify the following parts of the cricoid cartilage.

(a)   **Lamina**

(b)　Arch

(c)　Articular Surfaces

c.　Epiglottis

Describe the following structures in the spaces below.

(1)　Structure and Location

(2)　Attachments of the Epiglottis

(3)　Glossoepiglottic Folds

(a)　Epiglottic Valleculae

(b)　Laryngeal inlet

(4)　Epiglottitis

Why is epiglottitis a life-threatening condition?

2.   **Paired Cartilages of the Larynx**

a.   **Arytenoid Cartilages**

(1)   **Structure**

Describe the structure and the following aspects of the arytenoid cartilages.

(a)   **Vocal Processes**

(b)   **Muscular Processes**

(2)   **Function**

Describe the cricoarytenoid joint. What type of joint is it?

(a)   **Adduction/Abduction**

Describe the following movements of the arytenoid cartilages.

i)   **Rotation**

ii)   **Gliding or Sliding**

iii)   **Tilting**

(b) **Cartilaginous Glottis**

How much of the glottis is bordered by tissue with underlying cartilage? What are the physiological implications of this fact?

(c) **Membranous Glottis**

Why is the membranous glottis important in phonation?

b. **Minor Paired Cartilages of the Larynx**

Describe the locations of these minor cartilages.

(1) **Corniculate Cartilages**

(2) **Cuneiform Cartilages**

(3) **Triticeal Cartilages**

C. **Ligaments of the Larynx**

Describe the attachments of each of these ligaments. What are their functions? What differentiates an intrinsic ligament from an extrinsic ligament?

1. **Extrinsic Ligaments**

a. **Thyrohyoid Ligament**

    b.   Cricotracheal Ligament

2.   Intrinsic Ligaments

    a.   Conus Elasticus (Cricovocal Membrane)

    b.   Vocal Ligament

Describe the vocal ligament. What are its anterior and posterior attachments? How does it relate to the crico-vocal membrane?

    c.   Cricothyroid Ligament

Why is the cricothyroid ligament called the most important intrinsic ligament?

    d.   Vestibular Ligament

III.   Articulations of the Larynx

    A.   Cricothyroid Articulation

Describe the articulation of the thyroid cartilage with the cricoid cartilage.

     1.   Rotation About the Horizontal Axis

          What effect does this motion have on the pitch of the voice?

     2.   Gliding

B.   Cricoarytenoid Articulation

     Review cricoarytenoid articulation.

     1.   Rotation

     2.   Gliding or Sliding (Anterior/Posterior and Lateral/Medial)

     3.   Tilting

IV.   Cavities of the Larynx (Laryngopharynx)

     Describe these divisions of the laryngopharynx in relationship to one another.

     A.   Vestibular (Superior) Division

          1.   Location and Extent

          2.   Epiglottis

3.   **Aryepiglottic Folds**

Draw a diagram representing the cross-section of the laryngeal cavity in the box provided.

B.   **Ventricular (Middle Division)**

1.   **Location and Extent**

2.   **Ventricular Folds**

Is it possible to adduct the ventricular folds?

a.   **Composition**

b.   **Attachments**

3.   **Vocal Folds**

Describe the following aspects of the vocal folds. Why are these folds called the true vocal folds?

a.   **Composition**

(1)   **Thyroarytenoid Muscles**

(2)   Vocalis Muscles

(3)   Vocal Ligaments

(4)   Soft Tissue Layers

b.   Attachments and Positioning of the Vocal Folds

4.   Glottis

Draw a diagram of the glottis as seen from above. Show which part is intercartilaginous.

a.   Intermembranous

b.   Intercartilaginous

C.   Infraglottic (Subglottic) Division

What is the relationship of subglottic air pressure to voice loudness?

V.   Muscles of the Larynx: Intrinsic and Extrinsic

    A.   Intrinsic Muscles of the Larynx

        Why are these muscles referred to as intrinsic? What is the general function of the intrinsic muscles of the larynx? Describe the origins/insertions and functions of these muscles in the spaces provided.

        1.   Muscles That Control Tension/Length of the Vocal Ligament

            a.   Cricothyroid

            b.   Thyroarytenoid

            c.   Vocalis

        2.   Muscles That Control Glottal Aperture

            a.   Posterior Cricoarytenoid

            b.   Lateral Cricoarytenoid

            c.   Transverse Arytenoid

       d.   Oblique Arytenoid

   3.   Muscles That Modify Laryngeal Inlet

       a.   Aryepiglottic

       b.   Thyroepiglottic

       c.   Ventricular

B.   **Extrinsic Muscles of the Larynx**

Why are these muscles described as extrinsic? How would you describe the general function of the extrinsic muscles of the larynx? Describe the origins, insertions, and functions of the extrinsic muscles in the spaces provided.

   1.   Suprahyoid Muscles

       a.   Digastric

       b.   Stylohyoid

    c.   Mylohyoid

    d.   Geniohyoid

    e.   Hyoglossus

2.   Infrahyoid

    a.   Sternohyoid

    b.   Omohyoid

    c.   Thyrohyoid

    d.   Sternothyroid

3.   Indirect Displacers of the Larynx

    a.   Palatopharyngeus

b.   **Stylopharyngeus**

c.   **Inferior Pharyngeal Constrictor**

1. What is the most important biological function of the larynx?

    _____

2. The trachea is _____ to the esophagus.

3. What is the secondary or overlaid function of the larynx?

    _____

4. Describe the voice in physiological terms.

    _____

5. The perceived pitch of the voice is related to

    _____.

6. The perceived loudness of the voice is related to what physiological

    phenomenon? _____

7. Describe the glottis. _____

8. The hyoid bone is classified as a part of the _____.

9. The largest cartilage of the larynx is the _____.

10. The lowest cartilage of the larynx is the _____.

11. The flat parts of the thyroid and cricoid cartilages are called the _____.

12. The laryngeal prominence marks location of the _____.

13. The cartilage that is shaped like a signet ring is the _____.

14. The vocal ligaments are attached posteriorly to what structures?

    _____

15. Movement of the vocal folds away from the midline is called _____.

16. The muscles that tense and lengthen the vocal ligaments are the

    a. posterior arytenoid muscles.

    b. suprahyoid muscles.

    c. transverse arytenoid and oblique arytenoid muscles.

    d. cricothyroid, thyroarytenoid, and vocalis muscles.

17. Which of the following muscles do *not* adduct the vocal folds?

    a. posterior cricoarytenoid muscles

    b. lateral cricoarytenoid muscles

    c. oblique arytenoid muscles

    d. transverse arytenoid muscle

18. The lateral and posterior cricoarytenoid muscles attach to the arytenoid cartilages at which structures? _____

19. During heavy breathing, the vocal folds what position do the vocal folds assume? _____

20. Of what kind of joint is the cricoarytenoid joint an example? _____

21. The upper free border of the cricothyroid membrane is called the _____.

22. What distinguishes the intrinsic muscles of the larynx from the extrinsic muscles?

    _____

23. Which muscle pair abducts the vocal ligaments? _____

24. What are the main functions of the extrinsic muscles of the larynx?

    _____

25. What term is used to describe the air pressure inferior to the adducted vocal folds? _____

26. What is the average glottal frequency in adult females? _____

27.   Describe the forces that, according to currently held theories, act to close the glottis during phonation. _____

28.   Which muscles make up the vocal folds? _____ and _____

29.   In which direction does the thyroid cartilage move during deglutition (swallowing)? _____

30.   What role do the valleculae play in normal and disordered swallowing?

_____

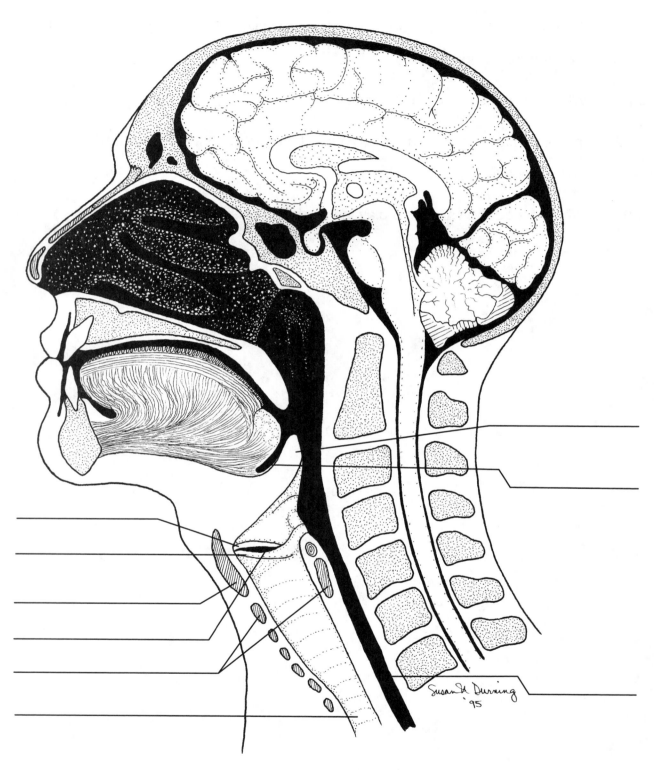

PHONATORY SYSTEM

92

SKELETON OF THE LARYNX

93

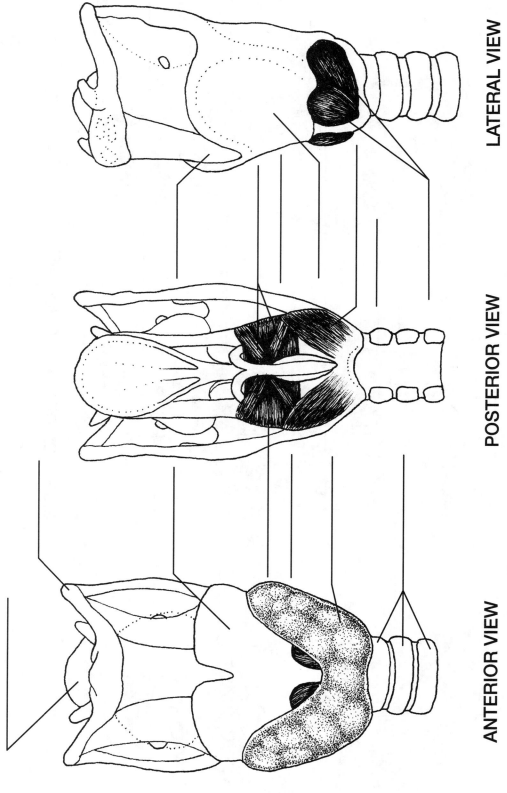

LATERAL VIEW

POSTERIOR VIEW

ANTERIOR VIEW

LARYNX

94

UNIT 5

THE ARTICULATORY MECHANISM

The primary functions of the articulatory structures are **mastication** (chewing), **deglutition** (swallowing), and **adjustment** of the opening of the airway and digestive tract entrance. The overlaid function of speech production is the result of millions of years of evolution. Human beings discovered that the extreme flexibility of their **branchial** musculature enabled them to produce a broad array of sounds when they moved in relationship to the less mobile structures of the upper airway.

To produce speech, the compressed air stream from the lungs, either voiced or unvoiced, is shaped by the muscles and structures of articulation as air leaves the system. Sounds produced this way are called **egressive**. Some languages employ sounds created by reversing the flow of air filling the lungs during speech, with the resulting sounds termed **ingressive**.

Speech is articulated through alteration of the shape of the **vocal tract**. The vocal tract is essentially a tube. It extends from the **glottis** to the openings of the nose and mouth. The structures that are used to alter vocal tract shape are referred to collectively as **articulators**.

Typically, the articulators are divided into fixed and mobile structures. The mobile structures move in relationship to the fixed ones, restricting air or altering the resonating characteristics of the tube of the vocal tract.

The **fixed articulators** are the **upper incisors, alveolar ridge** (superior), and the **hard palate**. The **upper incisors**, in combination with the tongue or lower lip, serve to create high-frequency consonants. The **hard palate**, formed by the maxillae and the palatine bones, separates the nasal and oral cavities. The anterior portion of the hard palate, from which the upper incisors erupt, is the **superior alveolar ridge**. This portion of the maxilla is so important to speech that it is usually considered a separate articulator. Since the inferior alveolar ridge is not used for standard speech articulation, the anatomical locator term is usually dropped. The fixed articulators provide a surface against which to juxtapose the tongue or lips for the alteration of resonance and the modification of airflow.

The mobile articulators are the **lips, mandible, velum, tongue, pharyngeal walls,** and **vocal folds**. The **lips** form a sphincter at the oral opening. They can occlude the oral cavity, articulate with the teeth, or form a ring through selective contraction of the **orbicularis oris** muscle. The formation of a labial ring serves as a fricative source or changes the resonance of the tract by extending its length and circular dimension. The **mandible** is mobile and adjusts the oral cavity opening by elevating and depressing. It works synergistically with the **tongue** to produce the fine adjustments necessary for vowel productions. The tongue is the most important structure of speech articulation. It is a flexible muscular structure covered with mucous membrane. Tongue muscles are divided into **extrinsic** and **intrinsic** groups. Extrinsic muscles have one connection outside the tongue and intrinsic muscles have both origin and attachment within the tongue. They are primarily involved in shaping the tongue for movement of food and liquid. They also play an important role making the fine adjustments necessary for vowel and consonant productions. The **velum** is continuous with the hard palate and extends posteriorly. It is a movable structure that serves to couple or uncouple the nasal cavity with the rest of the vocal tract.

Movements of the structures of articulation produce vowels and consonants of language phonology. These may be described by the location or place of maximum vocal tract constriction and the **manner** in which the airstream is managed. A third descriptor is the presence or absence of **voicing**. Although all vowels are voiced, some consonants are not. Dynamic patterns of articulator movement, opening and closing the vocal tract in various manners and at various locations, produce the audible **syllables** of speech. Speech sounds may either form the nucleus of syllables or form syllable boundaries. The study of speech sounds is **phonetics**.

Accomplishment of the objectives of this unit should provide the student with a basis for understanding the structure and function of the orofacial mechanism and the oropharynx. Checking the boxes beside each goal will help the student mark progress toward that understanding.

1. Describe the general anatomy of the vocal tract.

2. Describe the functions of the structures of the vocal tract in speech and swallowing.

3. Name the bones of the skull.

4. Describe the major divisions of the bones of the skull.

5. Name the structures of speech articulation.

6. Differentiate between the fixed and the mobile speech articulators.

7. Identify the cavities of the vocal tract and name the structures in each that are essential to normal speech and swallowing.

8. Name the muscles of facial expression essential to speech articulation.

9. Name the oral and pharyngeal muscles essential to normal speech and swallowing.

10. Describe, in general, the changes associated with normal growth of the head.

11. Describe the stages of deglutition.

I.   General Structure and Function of the Vocal Tract.

    A.   Structure

    Briefly describe the locations of the following articulatory mechanism structures.

        1.   Oral Cavity

            a.   Tongue

            b.   Dental Arches

            c.   Hard Palate

            d.   Velum (Soft Palate)

        2.   Nasal Cavity

            a.   Nares

            b.   Choanae

   c. Septum

  3. Pharyngeal Cavity

   a. Laryngopharynx

   b. Oropharynx

   c. Nasopharynx

B. Function

Describe these functional aspects of the articulatory mechanism as they apply to speech and/or deglutition.

  1. **Plosive and Fricative Sources for Obstruent Consonants**

   How do the structures of the oral cavity function to create constrictions for these sources? Are all obstruent consonants formed by constriction in the oral cavity?

  2. **Analogy to Band-Pass Filter for Vowels and Semivowels**

   Provide an example of how the muscles of the articulatory mechanism modify the phonatory source.

3.   **General Function**

Describe the oral cavity as the entrance to the alimentary canal. Differentiate between the routes of passage and list the structures involved in transferring food to the stomach and air to the lungs.

II.   **The Skull in General**

Describe the following structures in the spaces provided.

A.   **Gross Structure**

1.   **Skull**

a.   **Cranium**

(1)   **Facial Skeleton**

(2)   **Calvaria**

b.   **Mandible**

c.   **Hyoid bone**

2.   Cavities of the Cranium

Describe the locations and contents of these cavities of the cranium.

a.   Cranial Cavity

b.   Orbits

c.   Nasal Cavity

B.   Bone Type

C.   Mechanical Stresses

III.   Superior Aspect of the Cranium

A.   Calvaria

What sections of the skull comprise the calvaria? Describe the locations of the following bones of the calvaria.

1.   Frontal Bone

2.   Temporal Bones

3.   Sphenoid Bone

4.   Parietal Bones

5.   Occipital Bone

B.   Sutures

What type of joint is a suture? How do these joints change as the individual develops? Describe the locations of the following sutures.

1.   Sagittal

2.   Coronal

3.   Bregma

4.   Lambdoidal

5.   Pterion (Squamosal)

IV.   Inferior Aspect of the Cranium

Describe the forms and locations of the following structures in the spaces provided.

A.   Anterior Section

  1.   Hard Palate

  Describe the functions of the hard palate in speech and in deglutition.

  a.   Maxillae

    (1)   Palatine Processes

    (2)   Superior Alveolar Processes

    (3)   Incisive Fossa

  b.   Palatine Bones

c.   **Superior Teeth**

Identify the following teeth. Which teeth are essential for articulation of dental phonemes? Draw and label the superior dental arch of an adult in the box provided.

(1)   **Incisors**

(2)   **Cuspids**

(3)   **Bicuspids**

(4)   **Molars**

2.   **Growth and Development of Teeth**

By what age should the teeth necessary for the articulation of dental consonants erupt?

a.   **Teeth Eruption**

Give the normal ages of eruption of the superior dentition.

b.   **Anomalies of Occlusion**

Define the following terms for dental occlusion anomalies.

(1)   **Axiversion**

(a)   Distoversion

(b)   Mesioversion

(2)   Infraversion

(3)   Supraversion

(4)   Torsiversion

B.   **Middle Section of the Skull**

Describe the sphenoid and occipital bones as structures of the middle, inferior aspect of the skull.

1.   **Nasopharynx**

Locate the nasopharynx with respect to the inferior aspect of the skull.

2.   **Sphenoid Bone**

a.   **Pterygoid Plates**

Describe the pterygoid plates of the sphenoid bone as points of attachment for pharyngeal muscles.

(1)   **Pterygoid Muscles**

Describe the mandibular movement associated with these muscles. Why is this movement important in mastication?

(2)   **Tensor Veli Palatini**

Describe the origins and insertions of this muscle. What role does it play in speech? Describe the hamular processes of the sphenoid bone.

3.   **Occipital Bone**

What portion of the occipital bone contributes to speech articulation?

C.   **Posterior Section of the Inferior Skull**

1.   **Occipital Bone**

Describe the form and function of the following landmarks of the occipital bone.

a.   **Foramen Magnum**

b.   **Occipital Condyles**

c.   **Hypoglossal Canals**

2. **Temporal Bones**

Describe the form and function of the following landmarks of the temporal bones in the spaces provided.

   a. **Squamous Portions**

   b. **Petrous Portions**

   (1) **Auditory Meatuses**

   (2) **Bony Labyrinths**

   (3) **Levator Veli Palatini**

   Describe the origins and insertions of this muscle. What role does it play in speech?

   c. **Mastoid Processes**

   What muscles attach bilaterally to the sternum, clavicle, and mastoid process?

   d. **Styloid Processes**

   What muscles attach to the styloid processes bilaterally?

e.   Jugular Foramina

Briefly describe the functions of the following.

(1)   Internal Jugular Veins

(2)   Glossopharyngeal Nerves

(3)   Vagus Nerves

(4)   Accessory Nerves

f.   Carotid Canals

Briefly describe the functions of the following.

(1)   Internal Carotid Arteries

(2)   Sympathetic Plexuses

V.   Anterior Aspect of the Skull

Describe the forms and functions of the structures of the anterior skull in the spaces provided.

A.   The Face

1.   Importance in Communication

a. Speech

Which facial structures are involved in speech?

b. Facial Expression

Of what importance is facial expression in communication?

2. Bones of the Face

Describe the locations of these bones of the face.

a. Frontal Bone

b. Maxillae

c. Zygomatic Bones

d. Nasal Bones

e. Mandible

3.   Landmarks of the Face

Write the locations of these facial landmarks in the spaces provided.

    a.   Frontal Eminences

    b.   Orbits

    c.   Nose

        (1)   Nares

        (2)   Nasal Septum

    d.   Philtrum

VI.   Lateral Aspect of the Skull

Describe these bones articulations and landmarks of the lateral aspect of the skull.

A.   Bones

    1.   Frontal Bone

2. Parietal Bone

3. Sphenoid Bone

4. Temporal Bone

   a. External Auditory Meatus

   b. Mastoid Process

   c. Styloid Process

5. Occipital Bone

B. Articulations

Describe the locations of the following articulations of the skull bones. Include the names of the bones involved.

1. Temporo-Zygomatic

2. Pterion

VII.   **The Mandible**

Describe these features of the mandible. Of what importance is the mandibular movement to normal speech?

A.   **Importance in Speech**

1.   **Tongue Elevation**

2.   **Opening of the Oral Cavity**

3.   **Point of Attachment for Muscles of Speech Articulation**

Identify the muscles of speech articulation that attach directly to the mandible.

a.   Muscles that insert on the *Interior* aspect of the Mandible

b.   Muscles that attach to the *External* aspect of the Mandible

B.   **Importance in Deglutition**

Describe the importance of the mandible to mastication.

1.   **Opening of the Oral Cavity**

2. Mastication

Identify the muscles of mastication that attach directly to the mandible.

C. Structure of the Mandible

Describe the structure of the mandible in the spaces below.

1. Corpus

a. Mental Symphysis and Protuberance

b. Inferior Alveolar Arch

Of what importance are the mandibular teeth to speech?

2. Ramus

a. Condylar Process

b. Temporomandibular Joint

Describe the origins and insertions of the muscles that elevate the mandible. Which muscles depress the mandible? When are they used?

       (1)   **Muscles of Mandibular Elevation**

       (2)   **Muscles of Mandibular Rotation and Protrusion**

       (3)   **Muscles of Mandibular Depression**

    c.   **Coronoid Process**

       What muscle attaches to the coronoid process?

    d.   **Angle of the Mandible**

       How does the angle of the mandible change as the individual develops?

VIII.   **The Speech Articulators**

    A.   **Overview**

       1.   **Form**

          Describe the structures and locations of the fixed and mobile speech articulators. State their roles in the production of specific obstruent consonants.

          a.   **Fixed Articulators**

             (1)   **Upper Incisors**

(2)   Superior Alveolar Ridge

(3)   Hard Palate (Maxillae)

b.   Mobile Articulators

(1)   Lips

(2)   Mandible

(3)   Soft Palate (Velum)

(4)   Tongue

(5)   Pharyngeal Walls

(6)   Larynx

2.   Function in Speech

Describe how the speech articulators perform the following functions in the production of phonemes. Review place and manner of phoneme articulation.

a.   Modulation of Airflow for Obstruent Consonant Articulation

b.   Alteration of Resonance for Vowel and Approximant Articulation

c.   Formation of Cul-de-Sac for Nasal Articulation

3.   Function in Deglutition

Describe how the orofacial muscles perform the following functions in the intake of food and liquid.

a.   Retention of Material in Oral Cavity

b.   Protection of Airway

c.   Sealing of Oral Cavity for Pressure Change

d.   Mastication

e.   Transfer of Bolus

B.   Oral Speech Articulators in Detail

Describe these details of the oral speech articulators in the spaces provided.

1.   Extraoral (Facial) Articulators

a.   Lips

Draw a picture of the lips and indicate the vermilion zone and philtrum.

(1)   Vermilion Zone

(2)   Philtrum ("Cupid's Bow")

(3)   Effects of Lip Rounding

What are the speech effects of lip rounding?

b.   Muscles of Facial Expression

Describe the origins and insertions of these muscles. Describe the effects of their contraction.

(1)   Sphincteric Muscles

(a)   Orbicularis Oris

    (b)   Orbicularis Oculi

(2)   Horizontal Muscles

    (a)   Buccinator

    (b)   Risorius

(3)   Angular Muscles

    (a)   Levator Labii Superiorus

    (b)   Levator Labii Superiorus Alaeque Nasi

    (c)   Zygomaticus Major

    (d)   Zygomaticus Minor

    (e)   Depressor Labii Inferiorus

(4)   Vertical Muscles

   (a)   Mentalis

   (b)   Depressor Anguli Oris

   (c)   Levator Anguli Oris

(5)   Parallel Muscles

   (a)   Incisivus Labi Superiorus

   (b)   Incisivus Labi Inferiorus

Draw lines representing the courses of the fibers of the muscles of facial expression in the box provided. Indicate the names of the muscles you are representing.

c. **Function of Extraoral Articulators**

(1) **Labial Consonants**

List the labial consonants using the International Phonetic Alphabet.

(2) **Rounded Vowels**

List the rounded vowels of American English. Is lip rounding associated with articulation of any consonants?

(3) **Gestural Communication**

What is the gestural function of the facial articulators?

(4) **Retention of Fluids**

d. **Motor Innervation**

What is the major peripheral (cranial) nerve through which motor innervation of these muscles is provided?

e. **Sensory Innervation**

Through which major peripheral (cranial) nerve are sensations of pain, temperature, and touch conveyed from the face to the central nervous system?

2. **Intraoral Articulators**

Describe the form and functions of the following intraoral structures. What are their roles in the articulation of speech?

a. **Roof of the Oral Cavity**

What are the possible effects of an unrepaired fistula (cleft) of the roof of the oral cavity?

(1) **Maxilla (Hard Palate)**

(a) **Tissue Type**

(b)   Superior Alveolar Ridge

(c)   Upper Dental Arch

(2)   Velum (Soft Palate)

(a)   Uvula

(b)   Velopharyngeal Sphincter

      i)   Muscles of the Velopharyngeal Sphincter

      Describe the origins and insertions of the following muscles.

        a)   Tensor Veli Palatini

        b)   Levator Veli Palatini

        c)   Palatopharyngeus

d) **Palatoglossus**

e) **Superior Pharyngeal Constrictor**

ii) **Function of the Velopharyngeal Sphincter**

iii) **Motor Innervation**

Which peripheral nerves convey motor impulses from the central nervous system to the velopharyngeal sphincter muscles?

Draw a schematic representation of midsagittal view of the oral cavity in the box above. Include the lips, tongue, upper teeth, and the velum.

Draw a schematic representation of the open oral cavity as seen from the anterior aspect. Include the lips, tongue, upper teeth, and the velum.

b.   **Floor of the Oral Cavity**

(1)   **The Tongue**

Describe the role of the tongue in the articulation of speech. List the consonants produced by articulation of the tongue with the other oral structures. Describe the role of the tongue in the articulation of vowels.

(a)   **Gross Structure of the Tongue**

Describe the following.

i)   **Parts of the Tongue**

a)   **Apex**

b)   **Dorsum**

c)   **Front**

d)   **Back**

e)   **Blade**

f)   **Root**

ii)   **Tissue Type of the Tongue**

iii)   **Landmarks of the Tongue**

In the box provided, draw the dorsum of the tongue and show the tip, blade, median, front and back sulcus, sulcus terminalis, and foramen cecum.

iv)   **Attachments of the Tongue**

v)   **Intrinsic Muscles of the Tongue**

Describe the course of the fibers of the following muscles.

   a)   Vertical

   b)   Transverse

   c)   Superior Longitudinal

   d)   Inferior Longitudinal

vi)   **Extrinsic Muscles of the Tongue**

Describe the origins and insertions of these muscles.

   a)   Genioglossus

b) Styloglossus

c) Hyoglossus

d) Palatoglossus

vii) **Motor Innervation of the Tongue**

What nerve provides lower motor innervation of the tongue muscles?

viii) **Sensory Innervation of the Tongue**

What is the role of the touch and stretch receptors of the tongue in the treatment of articulatory disorders? Do taste receptors have a role in the treatment of swallowing disorders?

a) Touch

b) Taste

c. **Posterior Oral Cavity**

Where are the following structures located?

(1) **Faucial Arches**

(a)   Palatoglossus

(b)   Palatopharyngeus

(c)   Tonsillar Fossa

(2)   Tonsils (Waldeyer's Ring)

Describe the locations of the tonsils listed below.

(a)   Palatine Tonsils

(b)   Pharyngeal (Adenoid)

(c)   Lingual

(d)   Functions

(e)   Relevance to Speech Pathology

(3)   **Posterior (Oro) Pharyngeal Wall**

What functions do the posterior oral and pharyngeal structures have in modifying the quality of the speech signal?

(a)   **Superior and Middle Pharyngeal Constrictors**

(b)   **Passavant's Pad**

d.   **Functions of Intraoral Articulators**

In the box provided, draw a midsagittal view of the oral cavity with the velopharyngeal sphincter closed. Show the tongue, velum, a palatine tonsil, pharyngeal tonsil, and lingual tonsil.

IX. Deglutition

    A. Three Stages of Deglutition

Describe the progress of a bolus of food during each of these stages of deglutition.

        1. Oral Stage (Voluntary)

            a. Preparation of the Bolus

            b. Elevation of Oral Floor

            c. Posterior Propulsion of Bolus

            d. Constriction of Posterior Oral Cavity

            e. Closing of Velopharyngeal Sphincter

        2. Pharyngeal Stage (Involuntary)

            a. Bolus Propulsion

            b. Approximation of Aryepiglottic Folds

     c.   Arytenoid Cartilages Drawn Superiorly and Anteriorly

     d.   Elevation of Larynx and Articulation of Epiglottis

3.   Esophageal Stage (Involuntary)

1. Which part of the skull includes the calvarium and the facial skeleton?

   _____

2. A person viewing the skull from the lateral aspect would see which bones?

   _____

3. The cheeks are formed by which bones? _____

4. The mental protuberance is part of which bone? _____

5. What are the three cavities of the vocal tract? _____, _____,

   and _____.

6. Name the cavities of the cranium. _____

7. The frontal bone forms which facial structure? _____

8. Which muscles elevate the posterior part of the tongue? _____

9. Which of the following are *mobile* articulators?

   a) Tongue   b) Teeth   c) Alveolar Ridge   d) Velum   e) Lips

10. A fistula between the oral and nasal cavities is commonly called a _____.

11. Which facial muscle(s) contract(s) when the speaker forms /u/?

    _____

12. Which stage of deglutition is voluntary? _____

13. Which muscles contract to elevate the mandible? _____

14. Which articulators must function to produce /s/? _____

15. Describe the changes to the angle of the mandible that are coincident with aging.

    _____

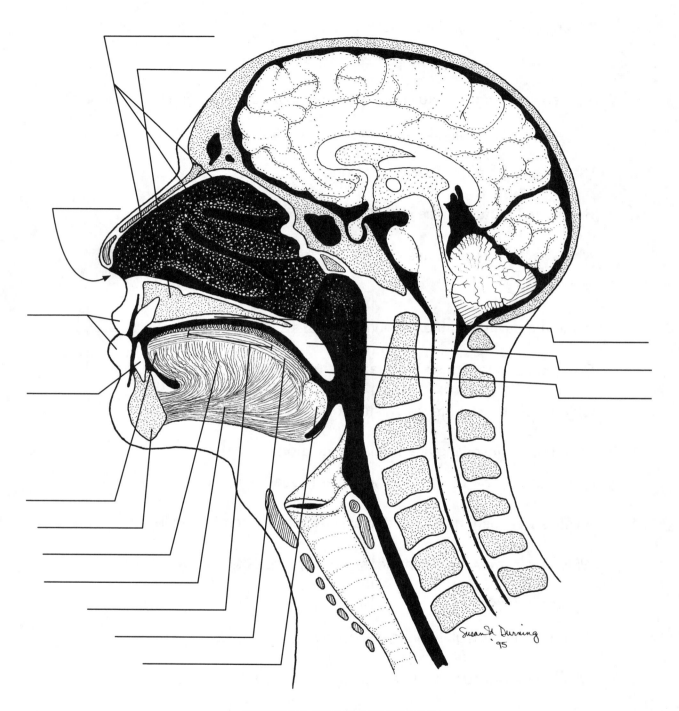

ARTICULATORY SYSTEM

136

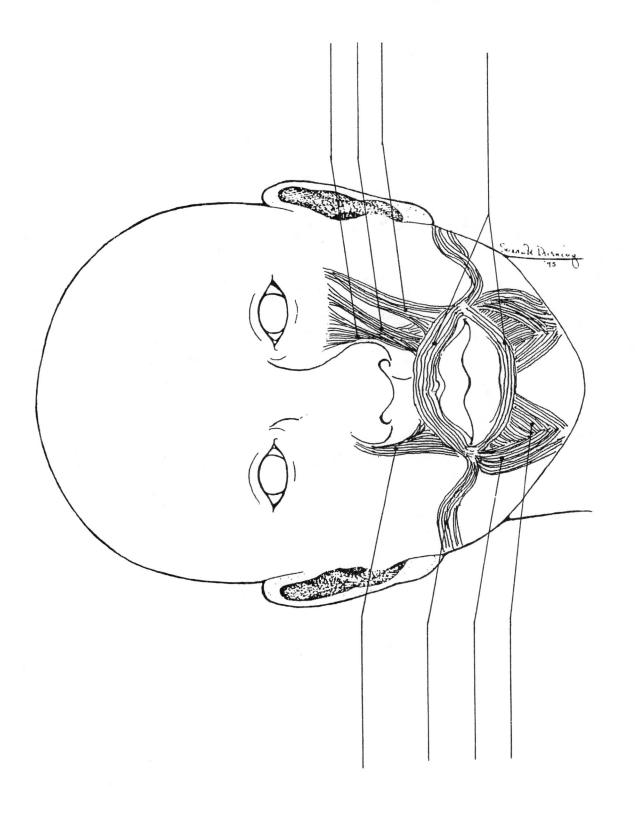

MUSCLES OF FACIAL EXPRESSION

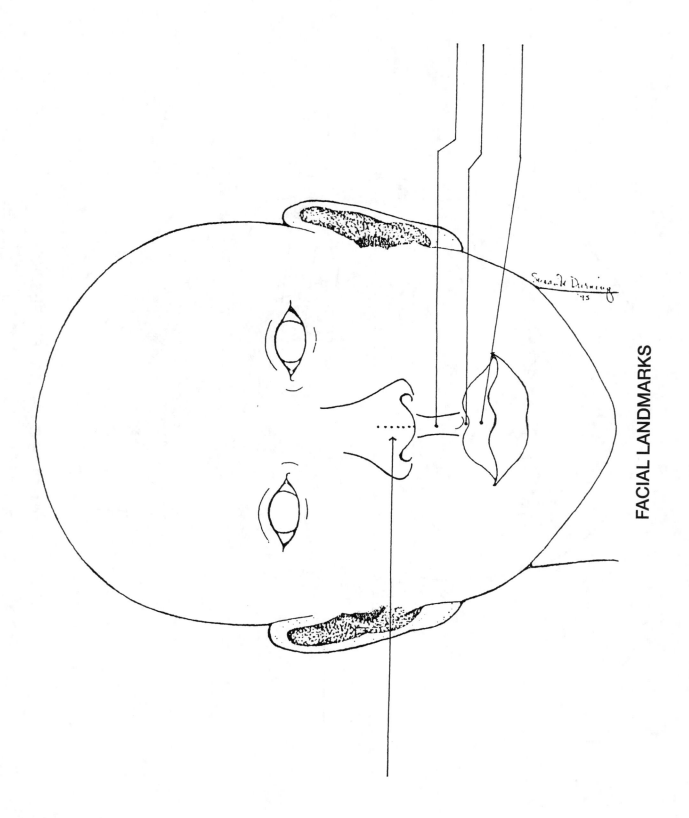

FACIAL LANDMARKS

138

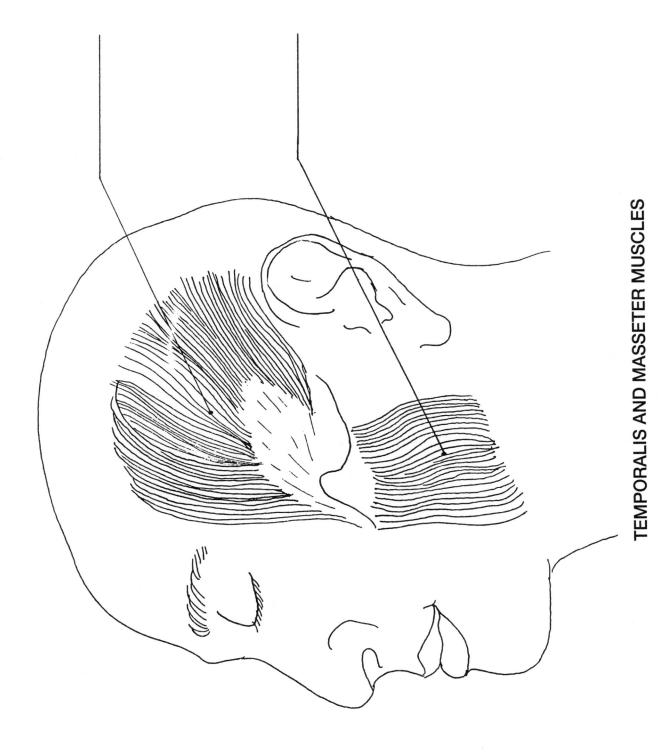

UNIT 6

THE NERVOUS SYSTEM

The nervous system is the medium by which the body realizes its wants and needs. Acting in concert with the endocrine system, the nervous system serves its function by virtue of the special conductivity and directionality of its constituent nervous tissue. The basic structure of the nervous system consists of the functional **neuron** and supportive **glial** tissues. The neuron consists of the **cell body** (soma), **axon, dendrite,** and the **synaptic junction**. It propagates ionic changes, called action potentials or neural impulses. These changes travel from the dendrites, past the cell body, to the axon. From there, they cross the cleft of the synapse to the next dendrite. Anatomists divide the nervous system into central and peripheral systems, but these divisions are for convenience only. The nervous system functions as a whole.

The central nervous system consists of the **brain** and **spinal cord**. Both are contained in the axial skeleton, and are covered by three membranes, the meninges. The central nervous system mediates input from the peripheral nerves and affects its responses through them.

The brain is divided into two **hemispheres** connected by the **corpus callosum** and other commissures. It contains more than 20 billion nerve cells and exercises executive control over higher mental sensory and motor functions. **Motor** and **sensory** functions of the right hemisphere are responsible for voluntary control and sensation on the left side of the body and vice versa. A **dominant hemisphere**, usually the left hemisphere, performs the crucial role in the reception and expression of language.

The gray **cerebral cortex** is a thin layer of cells covering the surface of the brain. It is a **convoluted** structure with **gyri** (ridges) and **sulci** (valleys) that serve as major anatomical landmarks for anatomists. Major sulci of the cortex include the **longitudinal, lateral,** and **central** sulci. The major gyri of the cerebral cortex include the **precentral, postcentral, angular, supramarginal gyri,** and the **pars triangularis**. **Broca's** and **Wernicke's** areas are the major expressive and receptive speech and language centers, working in concert to perceive, formulate, express, and monitor spoken language.

There are four **lobes** of the cerebral cortex named after the bones of the skull under which they are located: **frontal, parietal, temporal,** and **occipital**. The neuronal tissues of all the cerebral lobes receive, relay, reverberate, store, and retrieve impulses from external and internal sources. None function as an independent unit. The personality of an individual is the result of the combined functioning of all parts of the nervous system. The frontal lobe is the largest and forms the anterior portion of the hemisphere. The **motor cortex** and Broca's area are located in the frontal lobe. The **fissure of Rolando** or **central sulcus** divides the frontal and parietal lobes. The **primary motor cortex** lies immediately anteriorly to the central sulcus and the **primary sensory cortex** is posterior to this major landmark. The parietal lobe, forming the superior lateral portion of the hemisphere, is associated with the interpretation of somatosensory information. The **angular** and **supramarginal** gyri are also located in the area between the parietal and temporal lobes. These gyri are associated with the interpretation of symbolic stimuli. The temporal lobe comprises the inferior lateral section of the hemisphere. It is associated with the interpretation of auditory input. The **auditory cortex** or **Heschl's gyrus** is located in the temporal lobe. The **fissure of Sylvius**, or **lateral sulcus**, separates the temporal and frontal lobes. At the posterior region of the brain, the occipital lobe is delineated by the **parieto-occipital sulci**, visible on the medial surfaces of the hemispheres. The **primary visual cortex** is found in the occipital lobe. The **insular cortex** is sometimes identified as a cerebral lobe. It is located deep to the lateral fissure and is only visible by separating the bordering cortical tissue.

The interior of the brain contains the **white matter** and is made up of **afferent** and **efferent projection** fibers. White fibers are so called because they are sheathed in a white fatty **myelin sheath**. They converge at the **internal capsules** and **thalami** of each hemisphere, and descend through the **midbrain, pons,** and **medulla** levels of the **brainstem**. The white matter also contains **commissural** and **association** fibers that connect centers within and between the cerebral hemispheres.

Four **ventricles**, cavities filled with **cerebrospinal** fluid, are deep within the white matter. Cerebrospinal fluid is created in these ventricles and flows out and around the central nervous system. The fluid protects the central nervous system and helps regulate intracranial pressure.

The circulation of blood is critical to brain function. Neuronal tissues die very shortly after interruption in their ability to perform metabolism. Central nervous system neurons have very limited regenerative ability and are generally replaced with structural **glial** tissue after they die. The **internal carotid** and **vertebral arteries** supply blood to the brain. They conjoin at the **circle of Willis** where **anterior, posterior,** and **middle** cerebral arteries provide the primary blood supply to the hemispheres. Venous drainage is provided by the **dural sinuses** and the **jugular veins**.

The **spinal cord** is the caudal extension of the brainstem. It is the major conduit for impulses passing to or from the central nervous system. The spinal cord, as a central nervous system structure, processes some reflexive neural information. Spinal cord functions are said to be **segmental**.

The peripheral nervous system consists of the **12 cranial nerves, 31 spinal nerves,** and the **autonomic nervous system.** The cranial nerves have synaptic connections with the brainstem. They are final common pathways for most of the sensory and motor functions of the peripheral speech and hearing mechanisms. Spinal nerves synapse at nuclei at or very close to the spinal cord. The autonomic nervous system has both **sympathetic** and **parasympathetic** divisions that maintain and regulate unconscious bodily functions or adapt them in emergencies.

The objectives for this unit are to provide the student a foundation upon which to base further study of this vastly complex subject. Students should mark progress by checking the boxes beside each objective as they accomplish them.

✐ ☐ 1. Describe the general organization of the human nervous system.

✐ ☐ 2. Differentiate between afferent and efferent functions.

✐ ☐ 3. Describe the major components of the central nervous system.

✐ ☐ 4. Name the major parts of the human brain.

✐ ☐ 5. Name and describe the general functions of the lobes of the cerebral cortex.

✐ ☐ 6. Identify, using diagrams or models, the major landmarks of the cerebral cortex and describe their general functions.

✐ ☐ 7. Identify, using diagrams, the major subcortical structures of the brain and describe their major functions.

✐ ☐ 8. Identify and describe the general function of the cerebellum.

✐ ☐ 9. Name and describe the three meninges and their relative locations.

✐ ☐ 10. Describe the flow of cerebrospinal fluid.

✐ ☐ 11. Describe the major components of the peripheral nervous system.

✐ ☐ 12. Name and describe the communication functions of the cranial nerves.

✐ ☐ 13. Name and describe some commonly encountered syndromes associated with disorders of the human nervous system.

I.   General Organization of the Human Nervous System

Describe the overall organization of the human nervous system. How do the two major divisions serve each other? Is it realistic to consider the system as composed of two separate entities?

   A.   Basic Structures

   Describe the functional roles of neurons and glial cells. Describe the parts of a neuron.

      1.   The Neuron

         a.   Cell Body

         b.   Axon

         c.   Dendrite

         d.   Synapses

      2.   Glial Tissue

B.   Central Nervous System

Describe the locations and general functions of the major parts of the central nervous system.

    1.   Brain

         a.   Cerebral Hemispheres

            (1)   Cerebral Cortex

                (a)   Location

                (b)   General Function

            (2)   Subcortical Structures

                (a)   Location

                (b)   General Function

         b.   Brainstem

            (1)   Location

            (2)   General Function

      c.   Cerebellum

            (1)   Location

            (2)   General Function

  2.   Spinal Cord

      a.   Location

      b.   General Function

C.   Peripheral Nervous System

  1.   Spinal and Cranial Nerves

Give the general locations of the nuclei of the cranial and the spinal nerves. Describe the general differences in functions between cranial nerves and spinal nerves.

      a.   12 Cranial Nerves

      b.   31 Spinal Nerves

2. **Autonomic Nervous System**

   Describe the general differences between the sympathetic and parasympathetic divisions of the autonomic nervous system

   a. **Sympathetic Division**

   b. **Parasympathetic Division**

II. **Central Nervous System**

   A. **The Brain in Detail**

      Describe the form and functions of these structures of the brain.

      1. **Cerebral Hemispheres**

         a. **Cerebral Cortex**

            (1) **Structure of the Cerebral Cortex**

               (a) **Major Sulci of the Cerebral Cortex**

                  i) **Longitudinal Fissure**

                  ii) **Lateral Sulcus (Fissure of Sylvius)**

                  iii) **Insula**

iv)   Opercula

v)   Parallel Sulcus

(b)   **Central Sulcus (Fissure of Rolando)**

i)   Location of the Central Sulcus

ii)   Precentral and Postcentral Functions

(c)   **Major Gyri of the Cerebral Cortex**

Describe the locations of these gyri of the cerebral cortex.

i)   Precentral Gyrus

ii)   Postcentral Gyrus

iii)   Angular Gyrus

iv)   Supramarginal Gyrus

v)   Pars Triangularis

(2)   **General Functions of Areas of the Cerebral Cortex**

Describe the locations of these specific areas of the cerebral cortex. Draw their locations in the box provided.

(a)   **Sensory Cortex**

(b)   **Motor Cortex**

(c)   **Auditory Cortex**

(d)   **Visual Cortex**

2.   General Hemispheric Functions

    a.   Interhemispheric Differences

        (1)   Cerebral Dominance

        What is meant by cerebral dominance?

            (a)   Incidence of Left or Right Hemisphere Dominance

            (b)   Relationship to Handedness

        (2)   Dominant Hemisphere Functions

        (3)   Non-Dominant Hemisphere Functions

    b.   *Inter*hemispheric Communication

    Name and locate the major interhemispheric connections.

    c.   *Intra*hemispheric Communication

    Name and locate the major intrahemispheric communication pathways.

3. **Lobes of the Cerebral Cortex**

   Describe the forms and functions of the following structures.

   a. **Frontal Lobe**

      (1) **Location**

      (2) **Functions of the Frontal Lobe**

      Describe and name the possible effects of a lesion in the following locations.

      (a) **Motor Cortex (Precentral Gyrus)**

         i) **Homunculus (Projections)**

         ii) **Decussation of Motor Tracts**

      (b) **Association Areas**

         i) **Premotor Cortex**

         ii) **Broca's Area (Pars Triangularis)**

(c)   Other Functions

b.   Parietal Lobe

(1)   Location

(a)   Postcentral Gyrus

(b)   Somesthetic Cortex (Sensory Cortex)

(2)   Functions

Describe the possible effects of a lesion in the following locations.

(a)   Sensory Decussation

(b)   Sensory Homunculus

(c)   Stereognosis

Define stereognosis. What role does stereognosis play in the production (or perception) of speech?

(3)   **Angular Gyrus**

What effect might a lesion in this area have on communication?

(4)   **Supramarginal Gyrus**

What effect might a lesion in this area have on communication?

c.   **Temporal Lobe**

(1)   **Location**

(a)   **Temporal Gyri**

(b)   **Auditory Cortex (Heschl's Gyri)**

(2)   **Functions**

Describe and name the possible effects of a temporal lobe lesion on the following functions.

(a)   **Sensation (Reception)**

(b)   **Perception**

        (c)   Association

    (3)   Wernicke's Area

        Describe where this area is located and explain the potential effects on communication with a lesion in this area.

d.   **Occipital Lobe**

    (1)   Location

        (a)   Parieto-occipital Fissure

        (b)   Calcarine Fissure

        (c)   Visual Cortex

    (2)   Functions

        Describe and name the possible effects of a lesion on the following occipital lobe functions.

        (a)   Sensation

        i)   **Retinal Projections**

        ii)   **Optic Decussation**

        What is a "decussation?" Be alert for other examples of decussation in the central nervous system.

        iii)   **Anopsia**

        (b)   **Perception**

        (c)   **Association**

4.   **Subcortical Structures**

Describe the locations and functions of these subcortical structures in the spaces provided. Indicate the structures for which researchers have yet to reveal clear roles. Describe the possible effects of lesions in the following areas.

    a.   **Thalamus**

        (1)   **Location**

        (2)   **Structure**

(3)   Function

b.   Hypothalamus

c.   Pineal Body

d.   Basal Nuclei (Striate Bodies)

(1)   Names

(2)   General Location

(3)   Structure

(4)   Functions
What effect might a lesion in this area have on communication?

5.   **Brainstem**

Draw a schematic representation of the brainstem and label the three major divisions.

    a.   **Location**

        (1)   **Midbrain**

        (2)   **Pons**

        (3)   **Medulla**

    b.   **Relationship to Spinal Cord**

    c.   **Functions**

Briefly describe these central nervous system functions aggregated in the brainstem.

        (1)   **Ascending/Descending Tracts (CNS)**

            (a)   **Motor**

                i)   **Pyramidal**

                ii)   **Extrapyramidal**

(b)   Sensory

       i)   Spinothalamic Tracts

       ii)   Trigeminothalamic Tracts

       iii)   Posterior Column Lemniscal Tracts

(c)   Decussations

(d)   Reticular System

(e)   Vestibular System

6.   Cerebellum

a.   Location

b.   Function

7.   Meninges

    a.   Dura

    b.   Arachnoid

    c.   Pia

8.   Cerebrospinal Fluid (CSF)

    a.   Composition

    Describe the composition of cerebrospinal fluid.

    b.   Function

    What are the functions of cerebrospinal fluid?

    c.   Ventricles

    Where are the four ventriicles?

    d.   Foramina

    How does CSF flow from one ventricle to another?

e.   Subarachnoid Space

f.   Flow of Cerebrospinal Fluid

Describe the production, flow, and absorption of CSF.

B.   Spinal Cord in Detail

1.   Structure

Describe the sections of the spinal cord.

2.   Function

What is the function of the spinal cord?

III.   Peripheral Nervous System

A.   Spinal and Cranial Nerves

Describe the differences in locations and functions between the cranial nerves and the spinal nerves.

1. 12 Cranial Nerves

Beside each cranial nerve name, write its communicative function(s). Use the letters "S," "M," or "B" to indicate if the nerve has "sensory," "motor," or "both" functions.

Cranial Nerve	Communicative Functions	S/M/B
I Olfactory		
II Optic		
III Oculomotor		
IV Trochlear		
V Trigeminal		
VI Abducens		
VII Facial		
VIII Vestibulocochlear		
IX Glossopharyngeal		
X Vagus		
XI Accessory		
XII Hypoglossal		

2.   31 Spinal Nerves

Where are the spinal nerves located? What communicative functions do the spinal nerves perform?

B.   Autonomic Nervous System (Ganglia and Nerve Processes)

Describe the general differences between the sympathetic and parasympathetic divisions of the autonomic nervous system

1.   Sympathetic

a.   Thoracolumbar Outflow

b.   Emergency Actions

2.   Parasympathetic

a.   Craniosacral Outflow

b.   Normal Bodily Functions

1. What are the two main divisions of the human nervous system?

    _____ and _____

2. The central nervous system is composed of _____ and _____.

3. Sensory input is carried over _____ tracts.

4. Motor impulses are carried over _____ tracts.

5. The primary motor cortex is located in the _____ lobe.

6. There are _____ pairs of cranial nerves.

7. The spinal nerves are parts of the _____ nervous system.

8. The peripheral nervous system is subdivided into which parts?

    _____

9. The emergency acceleration in heart rate and increased perspiration which accompanies the presence of anxiety evoking stimuli is accomplished through action of _____.

10. The recognition that the (above) anxiety evoking stimuli are present is mediated by _____.

11. Nerves connect to one another at _____.

12. The raised portions of the convoluted surface of the cerebral hemispheres are called _____.

13. The temporal lobe is separated from the parietal and frontal lobes by _____.

14. The precentral and postcentral gyri are separated by _____.

15. The gyrus immediately posterior to the central sulcus is attributed with the function of _____.

16. Broca's area is located in the _____.

17. What condition will result when the visual cortex of one cerebral hemisphere is destroyed? _____.

18. A unilateral lesion of the motor cortex of the right hemisphere will result in _____.

19. The midbrain, pons, and medulla are parts of the _____.

20. The intrinsic muscles of the tongue receive their motor innervation via which cranial nerve? _____

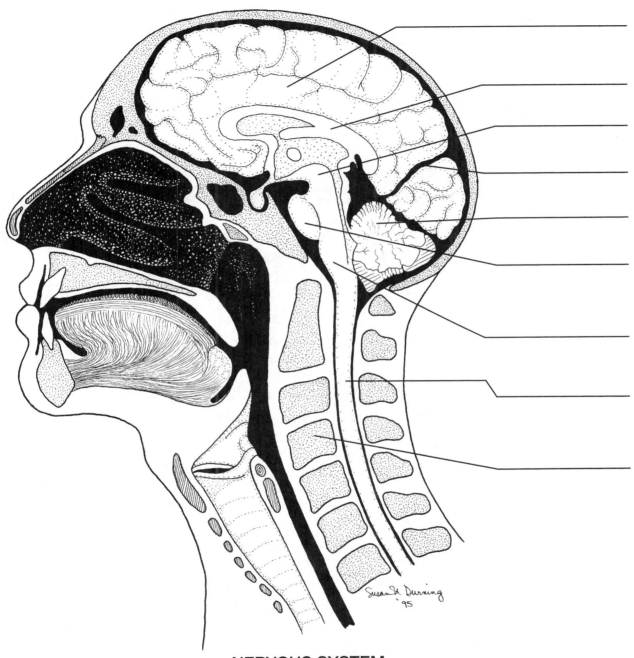

NERVOUS SYSTEM

UNIT 7

THE AUDITORY SYSTEM

The process of hearing depends on the transmission and transformation of energy. **Acoustic** energy must pass through three media and be converted into the **electro-chemical** energy of the nervous system before the listener becomes aware of its presence. The clarity with which the sound will be heard will depend upon the successful transmission of vibration energy from air to body tissues, and then to fluid.

Sound begins as the disruption of random molecular movements in a **medium**, usually air, by the directed displacements of a vibrating body. The vibrating body is referred to as the **source**.

Molecules in all matter are simultaneously attracted to and repelled from one another by the atomic forces of their components. The source applies additional force to adjacent molecules, and a chain reaction begins. Thus, the sound is **propagated**. Each displaced molecule in the medium absorbs some of the energy exerted upon it, but passes the residual energy on to the ones nearby. The process by which the molecules approach each other and bounce back is known as **compression** and **rarefaction.** Compression occurs when the distance between molecules is decreased and rarefaction occurs when the distance between the molecules is greater than during the normal state.

The listener becomes aware of the presence of sound when air molecules near the ear are set into motion with characteristics resembling those of the source. The sound must be of sufficient strength, or **intensity**, and within the anatomically determined range of **frequencies** to be transmitted by the ear and detected by the brain.

The **pinna** channels acoustic energy into the middle ear. The **external auditory meatus**, in its normal anatomical form, enhances sounds within the acoustic range of speech, and protects the sensitive deep structures of the auditory system. The external meatus leads to the **tympanic membrane**. The tympanic membrane divides the **outer** and **middle ear** and vibrates at a frequency and amplitude corresponding to the molecular displacements in the external meatus.

Sound energy passes on to the **middle ear**, or **tympanum**. The middle ear is an aspirin-sized cavity in the temporal bones of the skull. Since the cavity is closed at each end, a **eustachian tube** passes from within to the nasopharynx. This tube serves to equalize air pressure when required. Secured to the tympanic membrane are the three tiny bones of the middle ear known as the **ossicles: malleus, incus,** and **stapes**. These bones vibrate in unison with the tympanic membrane and amplify the energy transmitted to the inner ear.

The **inner ear** contains the sensory end organ of hearing, the **cochlea**. The cochlea is part of a complex sensory structure called the **labyrinth**. The labyrinth is so named because it consists of soft tissue organs embedded in a series of tunnels hollowed out of the temporal bone of the skull. The cochlear tunnel is snail-shaped. Here, the medium of sound transmission becomes a fluid called **endolymph**. The fluid within the cochlea is set into vibration, which in turn, sets the **organ of Corti** on the **basilar membrane** into vibration. This vibration occurs at a frequency and amplitude corresponding to the ossicular chain vibration. Attached to the organ of corti are epithelial stereocilia, or **"hair cells,"** connected to the nerve endings of the **spiral ganglion**. Each hair cell movement sets off a subsequent neurological impulse along the **vestibulocochlear** or **eighth cranial nerve**. At this stage of the hearing process, the hydraulic energy occurring in the cochlea transforms into nerve or electrochemical energy.

The vestibulocochlear nerve enters the brainstem at a structure called the pons. From the pons, some nerve fibers enter a structure known as the **thalamus.** It is the thalamus, in combination with other brain structures, that regulates which auditory signals are attended to and those to be ignored. From the thalamus, the electrochemical energy is transmitted upward to the cortex where interpretation of the sound occurs.

Another sensory structure of the labyrinth is the **vestibular system**. This system senses the pull of gravity on its receptors. Its nerve endings interact with the body's axial and appendicular skeletal muscles, and with the extraocular eye muscles. The vestibular system helps the body maintain its posture through the sense of balance. It consists of the **utricle**, the **saccule,** and three **semicircular canals**.

Objectives for this unit are intended to orient the student to the fundamental form and function of the auditory system. With such preparation, the student should be ready to pursue further study in audiology, speech-language pathology, or related fields. Students should check the boxes beside each objective to mark progress toward that overall goal.

1. Identify and describe the functions of the two main divisions of the human auditory system.

2. Describe the structures of the human auditory system as being located in the peripheral or central divisions of the auditory system.

3. Identify the anatomical limits and describe the functions of the peripheral hearing mechanism.

4. Name the three main parts of the peripheral hearing mechanism.

5. Describe the structures of the peripheral hearing mechanism as being located in the external, middle or inner ear(s).

6. Locate the major landmarks of the pinna.

7. Name and describe the morphologies and locations of the ossicles.

8. Describe the major functions of the parts of the peripheral hearing mechanism, including the:

   - Pinna
   - Ossicles
   - External Auditory Meatus
   - Cochlea
   - Tympanic Membrane
   - Vestibule
   - Tympanum
   - Semicircular Canals
   - Eustachian Tubes
   - Vestibulocochlear Nerve

9. Identify and describe the functions of the following structures of the cochlea:

   - Scala Media
   - Scala Tympani
   - Scala Vestibuli
   - Organ of Corti
   - Stereocilia
   - Auditory Nerve
   - Reissner's Membrane
   - Basilar Membrane
   - Tectorial Membrane
   - Endolymph
   - Perilymph
   - Helicotrema

✐ ☐ 10. Identify the anatomical limits and describe the functions of the central auditory system.

✐ ☐ 11. Describe, in sequence, the transmission of auditory evoked potentials with respect to the following central auditory system structures:

- Cochlear Nuclei
- Superior Olivary Complex
- Medial Geniculate Body of the Thalamus
- Cerebral Cortex

I.   Two Main Divisions of the Human Auditory System

Describe the location and functions of the two main divisions of the human auditory system.

    A.   Peripheral Auditory System

        1.   Location and Extent

        2.   Functions

    B.   Central Auditory System

        1.   Location and Extent

        2.   Functions

II.   The Peripheral Hearing Mechanism in Detail

Describe the forms (extent) and functions of the following structures of the peripheral hearing mechanism in the spaces provided.

A.   External (Outer) Ear

    1.   Pinna (Auricle)

        a.   Form

        Draw a pinna in the box provided. Locate the following parts and label them on your illustration.

          (1)   Helix

          (2)   Antihelix

          (3)   Tragus

          (4)   Antitragus

          (5)   Lobe

          (6)   Concha

          (7)   Triangular Fossa

        b.   Functions of the Pinna

        What are the hearing functions of the pinna? Does the pinna have functions other than those for hearing?

    2.   External Auditory Meatus

        a.   Form

(1)   Ear Canal

    (a)   Shape

    (b)   Underlying Tissue Composition

    (c)   Cerumen

        What are the origin and purposes of cerumen?

(2)   Tympanic Membrane

    Is the tympanic membrane part of the outer or middle ear? In the spaces below, describe the parts of the tympanic membrane and their functions.

    (a)   Laminae

    (b)   Pars Tensa

    (c)   Pars Flaccida

(d)   Otoscopic Landmarks

Draw a schematic representation of the tympanic membrane as seen from the external auditory meatus in the box provided. Label the following landmarks:

Pars Tensa

Pars Flaccida

Malleolar Stria

b.   Functions

Describe the functions of the external auditory meatus in the spaces provided.

(1)   Acoustic Function

(2)   Protective Function

c.   Mastoid Process (of Temporal bone)

How do audiologists use the mastoid process to specify the natures of hearing disorders?

B.   Middle Ear (Tympanum)

Describe these aspects of the middle ear in the spaces provided.

1.   General Form and Extent

2.   Function

3.   Structures of the Middle Ear

a.   Tympanic Membrane

(1)   Structure

Describe the laminae of the tympanic membrane.

(2)   Function

b.   Ossicles

(1)   Form

In the box provided, draw a stylized diagram of the relationship of the ossicular chain from the tympanic membrane to the oval window. Label each ossicle.

(a)   Malleus

(b)   Incus

(c)   Stapes

(2)   **Impedance Matching Function**

Describe two ways the ossicular chain matches acoustic impedance between the atmosphere and the cochlear fluids.

c.   **Eustachian (Pharyngotympanic) Tubes**

(1)   **Structure and Location**

(2)   **Function**

d.   **Muscles of the Middle Ear**

(1)   **Stapedius**

(2)   **Tensor Tympani**

      (3)   **Acoustic Reflex**

      Does the acoustic reflex serve a protective function?

4.   **Middle Ear Function Testing**

Describe how audiologists test the function of the middle ear. Why is the otoscope an important tool in the examination of the peripheral hearing mechanism?

C.   **Inner Ear (Labyrinth)**

1.   **Location**

In what portion of the temporal bone is the inner ear located?

2.   **Bony Labyrinth**

3.   **Membranous Labyrinth**

4.   **Inner Ear Structures**

     a.   **Hearing Mechanism**

      (1)   **Cochlea**

(a)   Shape

Describe the shape of the cochlea. How many turns does it make from basal to apical ends?

    i)   Basal End

    ii)   Apical End

(b)   Membranous Portion of the Cochlea

    i)   Scala Media

Where are these fluids found relative to the scala media?

        a)   Endolymph

        b)   Perilymph

    ii)   Basilar Membrane

Describe these structures of the basilar membrane.

        a)   Organ of Corti

       b)   Stereocilia (Hair Cells)

       c)   Tectorial Membrane

       d)   Spiral Ganglion

     iii)   Reissner's (Vestibular) Membrane

(c)   **Bony Portion of the Cochlea**

Describe the locations of these structures of the bony portion of the cochlea. What hearing function do these structures play?

    i)   Scala Tympani

    ii)   Scala Vestibuli

    iii)   Helicotrema

    iv)   Modiolus

(2) **Cochlear Nerve**

What is the other division of the eighth cranial nerve?

(a) **Cranial Nerve VIII: Auditory Division**

i) **Cochlear Nerve Nuclei**

ii) **Cochlear Nuclear Synapses**

b. **Vestibular Mechanism**

Describe these structures of the vestibular mechanism. What is the general function of this mechanism?

(1) **Utricle**

(2) **Saccule**

(3) **Central Structure of Labyrinth**

(4) **Semicircular Canals**

(a) **Vertical Canals**

(b)   Horizontal Canal

c.   Inner Ear Functions

(1)   Functions for Hearing Mechanism

(a)   Basilar Membrane

i)   Frequency Analysis

ii)   Transduction

How does the basilar membrane act as an energy transducer?

(b)   Auditory Nerve

i)   Threshold

Define threshold *as it applies to auditory testing.*

ii)   Firing Rate of the Nerve

How does firing rate of the auditory nerve relate to the listener's perception of loudness?

iii)   Frequency Perception

What is the current theory regarding the role of the auditory nerve in frequency perception?

iv)   Temporal Perception

What is meant by "temporal perception?"

(2)   Functions of Vestibular Mechanism

Describe the significance of these aspects of vestibular function.

(a)   Perception of Position in Space

(b)   Relationship to Extraocular Muscles

(c)   Relationship to Muscles of Posture and Locomotion

III.   The Central Auditory System

In the spaces provided, describe these anatomical aspects of the central auditory system.

A.   Location and Limits

B.   Structures of the Central Auditory System

    1.   Brainstem Structures

        a.   Pons

        b.   Midbrain

    2.   Thalamus

      What other special senses have relay centers in the thalamus?

    3.   Cerebral Cortex

        a.   Heschl's Gyrus

        b.   Association Areas

C.   Functions of the Central Auditory System: The Central Auditory Pathways

Describe the course of auditory stimuli from the cochlea to the cerebral cortex via the structures listed below. How are these action potentials tracked? How do audiologists employ such tracking for diagnostic purposes? Describe any role physiologists feel it may have in refining the listener's perception of auditory stimuli.

1.　Brainstem

    a.　Pons

        (1)　Cochlear Nuclei

            (a)　Dorsal Cochlear Nucleus

            (b)　Ventral Cochlear Nucleus

                i)　Anteroventral Cochlear Nucleus

                ii)　Posteroventral Cochlear Nucleus

            (c)　Tonotopic Representation

What is tonotopic representation?

        (2)　Superior Olivary Complex

            (a)　Decussation

            (b)　Localization of Sound Source

            (c)　Olivocochlear Tracts

b. Midbrain

    (1)   Lateral Lemniscus

        (a)   Inferior Colliculus

        (b)   Nucleus of the Lateral Lemniscus

        (c)   Olivocochlear Bundle Fibers

            How do audiologists use action potentials from the olivocochlear fibers to evaluate cochlear functions?

    (2)   Association with Other Functions

2.   Thalamus

    a.   Location

    b.   General Function

        (1)   Sensory

        (2)   Emotional

c.   **Medial Geniculate Body**

3.   **Cerebral Cortex**

Does the cerebral cortex appear to deal differently with meaningful auditory stimuli than it does with nonmeaningful ones?

a.   **Temporal Lobe**

(1)   **Heschl's Gyrus**

(2)   **Association Areas**

(3)   **Interaction with Other Cortical Functions**

Describe the way auditory signals are associated with signals from other input modalities at the level of the cerebral cortex.

b.   **Interhemispheric Differences**

(1)   **Sensation**

(2)   Perception

Describe what is meant by "perception." Are there different levels of perception?

    (a)   Perception of Speech

    (b)   Perception of Other Stimuli

(3)   Auditory Discrimination

    (a)   Of General Acoustic Stimuli

    (b)   Of Speech Stimuli

(4)   Auditory Memory

1.   The external auditory meatus is part of the _____.

2.   What is the major contribution of the pinna to hearing?

     _____

3.   The skeleton of the distal portion of the external auditory meatus is composed

     of _____.

4.   The main function of the middle ear is to _____.

5.   The ossicular chain is composed of which three bones?

     _____

6.   Pressure equalization for the middle ear is provided by

     _____.

7.   The semicircular canals are parts of the _____.

8.   The end organ for hearing is the _____.

9.   With what fluid are scala vestibuli and scala tympani filled? _____.

10. The cranial nerve which carries sound activated nerve impulses to the

     brainstem is _____.

11. The cranial nerves connect to the central nervous system at what structure?

     _____

12. Nerve fibers of the auditory pathways cross from one side of the brainstem to

     the contralateral side at the level of the _____.

13. In most people, meaningful language input is mediated primarily in the

     _____.

14. The auditory cortex is located in the _____.

15. The first synapses of the central auditory pathway are the

    _____.

16. A tumor that affects transmission of VIIIth nerve impulses is called

    _____.

17. Indicate in which division (central or peripheral) of the auditory system the following structures are located.

    a. stapedius muscle   _____

    b. cochlea   _____

    c. pinna   _____

    d. dorsal cochlear nucleus   _____

    e. inferior olive   _____

    f. stapes   _____

    g. ceruminous glands   _____

    h. VIIIth nerve   _____

    i. Heschl's gyrus   _____

    j. organ of Corti   _____

18. The semicircular canals are parts of what system? _____

19. Which ossicle is located closest to the tympanic membrane? _____

20. What are the three main parts of the peripheral hearing mechanism?

    _____

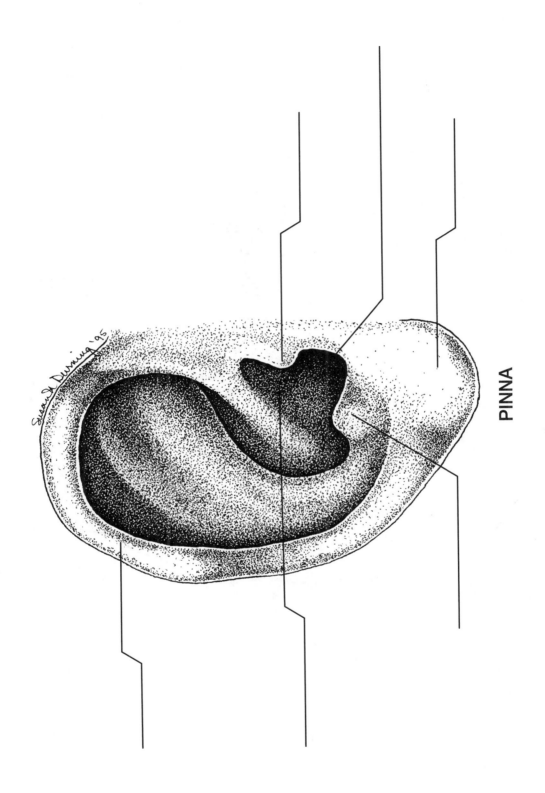

PINNA

197

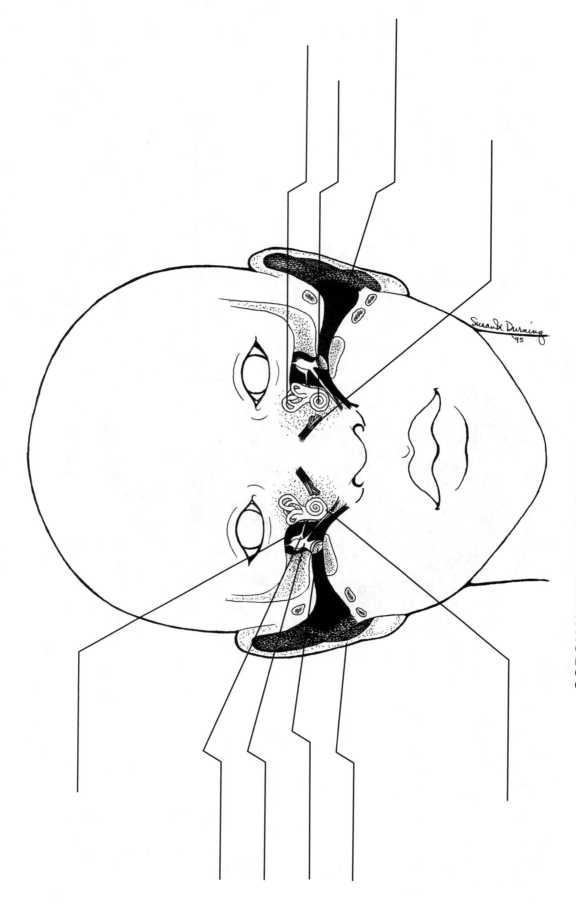

CORONAL VIEW OF PERIPHERAL HEARING MECHANISM

PART II
ACTIVE LEARNING GUIDE

The Active Learning Guide is provided in the second edition as one of several means for students to respond to items in the Study Outline units. It contains text and illustrations keyed to study outline items.

The authors urge students to use their textbooks and other referential materials in addition to the Active Learning Guide as a means to assimilate and master the basics of anatomy and physiology of speech and hearing. The use of multiple sources and repeated exposures reinforces learning and will lead students to our goal of practical application of the material.

UNIT 1

INTRODUCTION TO ANATOMY AND PHYSIOLOGY

I   Definitions

A.   **Anatomy**

Anatomy is the study of the structures of organisms and the relationship of their parts. The word "anatomy" is derived from the Greek language and originates from the words, "to cut up" (Zemlin, 1998).

B.   **Physiology**

Physiology is the study of the activities and functions of living organisms and their parts. The word "physiology" is derived from the Greek word, physis, which means "nature."

II.   Subdivisions of Anatomy

A.   **Descriptive Anatomy:** The branch of anatomy in which the body is considered as a number of systems, each of which consists of homogeneous tissue and has a certain functional unity.

B.   **Applied Anatomy:** The branch of anatomy concerned with the practical application of the study of the structures of the body to a specialized field (e.g., surgery).

C.   **Microscopic Anatomy:** The branch of anatomy concerned with the details of structure as revealed through a microscope (i.e., the study of cells and tissues).

D.   **Developmental Anatomy:** The study of the growth of the organism from the single cell to birth.

E.   **Geriatric Anatomy:** The study of the morphophysiology of the long-lived individual.

III.   Subdivisions of Physiology

A.   **General Physiology:** The science of general laws of life and functional activity. Relevance: A fundamental physiological law is that oxygen is required for animal cell metabolism. Therefore, airway patency is of paramount importance in treatment of swallowing disorders because the mechanics of respiration for life also apply to respiration for speech.

B.   **Applied Physiology:** The study of how the knowledge of physiology can be used to solve problems in medicine or industry. Relevance: Studies have determined that sustained, high ambient sound pressure levels cause permanent damage to the inner ear. This knowledge led to Occupational Safety and Health Association (OSHA)-mandated noise abatement programs in factories.

C. **Experimental Physiology:** Experimental physiology reveals information about the function of living organisms through the use of animal or human subjects. Relevance: Studies have determined that children have a fairly predictable ontogeny of speech development. Therefore, a clinician can place children in treatment with more confidence by comparing their speech performances with their chronologic ages.

D. **Special Physiology:** The study of the function of specific organs. For example, cardiology is the study of the heart, endocrinology is the study of organs that secrete internally, and neurology is the study of the nervous system. Relevance: Speech-language pathologists and audiologists use findings from the neurology branch of special physiology to understand the neural basis for speech, language, and hearing.

E. **Pathologic Physiology:** The study of functions that have been modified by disease processes. This field has primary relevance to speech-language pathologists who study disordered language and communication. Relevance: Laryngeal function can be severely compromised by the invasion of cancerous lesions. Speech-language pathologists must understand the course and nature of such damage to develop effective treatment programs.

IV. **Anatomical Position**

For descriptive purposes, a standard position and standard terms are used to allow a universal regional representation of the body. The anatomical locator terms used in this text, and in most other texts, are based on a standard anatomical position.

A. **Position**

1. Body Standing Erect

2. Face Forward

3. Arms Extended Downward at Sides

4. Palms Forward

B. **Names of Major Topographic Regions**

1. *Cranial Region:* extends from the top of the head to the bottom of the mandible and to the foramen magnum.

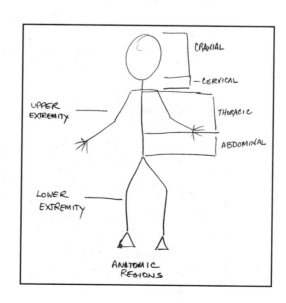

2. *Cervical Region:* extends from the foramen magnum to the thoracic inlet.

3. *Thoracic Region:* extends from the thoracic inlet to the diaphragm.

4. *Abdominal Region:* extends from the diaphragm to the pelvic floor.

5. *Upper Extremities:* extend from the clavicles and scapulae to the fingertips, including the shoulders, arms, forearms, wrists, hands, and fingers.

6. *Lower Extremities:* extend from the ilium to the toe tips, including the hips, thigh, legs, ankles, feet, and toes.

V. **Anatomical Planes of Reference**

A. **Sagittal:** Divides the body into right and left sections and runs parallel to the sagittal suture of the skull.

B. **Coronal:** Divides the body into anterior and posterior sections. Runs perpendicular to the sagittal plane.

C. **Transverse (Horizontal):** Divides the body into superior and inferior sections.

VI. **Anatomical Location Terms Presented as Antonyms (Opposites)**

Peripheral	Central
Toward the outer surface. The outer ear is peripheral to the inner ear.	Relating to the center. The brain is central to the skull.
Ventral	**Dorsal**
Toward the stomach or away from the backbone. The trachea is ventral to the esophagus.	Toward the backbone. The spine is dorsal to the stomach.
Anterior	**Posterior**
Toward the front. The toes are anterior to the heels.	Toward the back. The esophagus is posterior to the trachea.
Superficial	**Deep**
At the surface (distinct from "superior" because the surface might not be on top). The skin is superficial to the organs.	Away from the surface (distinct from "inferior"). The organs are deep in relation to the skin.

Superior	Inferior
Above. The head is superior to the torso.	Below. The knees are inferior to the hips.
Medial	**Lateral**
Toward the middle. The third finger is medial to the other fingers.	Toward the side. The ears are lateral to the skull.
Proximal	**Distal**
Toward the body or toward the oot of a free extremity. The shoulder is proximal in relation to the hand.	Away from the body or away from the root of a free extremity. The hand is distal to the elbow.
Caudal	**Rostral (Cranial)**
Toward the tail or away from the head. The brainsteam is caudal to the cerebral cortex.	Toward the nose or beak. The nose is rostral to the brain.
External	**Internal**
Outside; can be interchanged with superficial.	Inside; can be interchanged with deep.

UNIT 2

CYTOLOGY AND HISTOLOGY

I. **General Notes**

    A. **Cytology**

        The science of the study of cells is called cytology. Cells are the basic building blocks of the body.

    B. **Histology**

        The study of tissues is called histology. Tissues are collections of cells that have similar structure and function.

II. **Cytology**

    A. **Definition of the Cell**

        A cell is the smallest unit of life. It is the basic physiologic constituent of the body. All eukaryotic cells have an outer membrane called the plasma membrane which contains a substance called cytosol, a cytoskeleton, and several types of smaller subcellular entities called organelles.

    B. **Characteristics of Living Matter**

        1. *Characteristics of Life in All Organisms*

            a. *Growth:* Increase in size (length, weight, volume, etc.).

            b. *Reproduction:* The ability to produce new protoplasm or new offspring of the same type.

            c. *Metabolism:* The ability to convert food and oxygen into energy for maintenance of the cell's activities.

            d. *Adaptation or Irritability:* The capability to sense environmental changes and adjust to them.

        2. Characteristics of Life in Some Organisms

            a. *Spontaneous Movement:* Movement that originates within the organism. *Fungi do not exhibit spontaneous movements.*

            b. *Expression of Consciousness:* Ability to demonstrate awareness of reality. *Plants do not express consciousness.*

c.   *Voluntary Use of Senses:* Ability to orient sensory receptors to specific stimuli of interest. *Amoebas have no voluntary use of senses.*

C.   General Structure of the Cell

1.   **Protoplasm:** Protoplasm is the substance of all cells. This word comes from the Greek words for "first" and "thing that is formed." Two basic types of protoplasm found in a typical cell are cytoplasm, which forms the bulk of the cell's protoplasm and nucleoplasm, a thicker protoplasm contained in the nucleus.

2.   **Cytoplasm:** The cytoplasm is a thin substance that constitutes the outer part of the protoplasm. The cytoplasm contains a number of structures or organelles associated with synthesis of chemical substances, depending on the function of the individual cell. For example, mitochondria are responsible for making adenosine triphosphate (ATP), and centrosomes, associated with cell structure organization are found within the cytoplasm.

3.   **Nucleus:** The nucleus ("nut" or "kernel") is the largest of the organelles in the cytoplasm. It contains the genetic material (chromosomes) of the organism, and the centers for creating proteins (ribosomes).The cell nucleus is surrounded by a netlike supportive structure called the endoplasmic reticulum.

4.   **Cell Fluids:** Fluids fill and surround all the cells. The fluids are mostly (70–85%) water. Intracellular fluid is located inside the plasma membrane of each cell and is composed of water and proteins. Extracellular (or intercellular) fluid is located in the spaces between the cells.

5.   **Cell Shape:** Cell shape depends on the way the cells are grouped and the forces (stresses) that act on them. The cytoskeletal structure of the cell (cellulose fibers that form a kind of skeleton for the cell) also provide some cells with their unique shape. The shapes of the cells sometimes are the basis for the names of the tissues they comprise. For instance, cells forced into little cubes are called cuboidal cells. Flat cells are called squamous cells. Cells shaped like goblets are called goblet cells. There are about 100 trillion cells in the human body. Thus, cells are pretty small. Their size is measured in microns (1/1,000,000 meter). A red blood cell is about 7 to 8 microns in diameter. There are, however, some cells that are relatively large in size. Some nerve cells (neurons) can have fibers that are visible to the naked eye and are measured in meters.

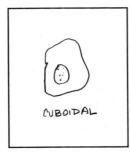

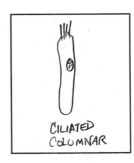

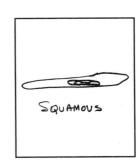

III.   Histology

A.   Definition of Tissue

An aggregation of cells organized to perform a specific bodily function is called a *tissue* (Culbertson & Tanner, 2011). There are several types of tissue, classified variously according to different anatomists. In general, tissues are classified according to the form or functions of their composite cells, and the nature of the material between the cells. Tissues can be classified embryologically (based on the germ layer from which it developed), structurally (based on its form or shape) or functionally (based on its role in the body physiologically).

B.   Four Basic Tissue Types

1.   *Epithelial*

- Epithelial tissues form the protective coverings of the body. This tissue type covers the face and hands, as well as the inside of the oral, nasal, and pharyngeal cavities.

- Epithelial tissue is distinguished from other tissues by its intercellular structure and its cellular arrangement. Epithelial tissue has very little material between the cells intercellular material or matrix); its cells are closely packed together. The cells of epithelial tissue are arranged in a flat or mosaic pattern. They also have a free surface, meaning that one end is not covered. The free end faces the outside of the body or the inside of a body cavity, such as the stomach. Epithelial cells are usually situated over a layer of connective tissue and are separated from it by a basement membrane, formed of structural substances secreted by the epithelial cells themselves.

2.   *Connective*

- Connective tissue is most distinguishable because of its great variability of intercellular structure. It has few cells and a great deal of material between these cells. This intercellular material is called matrix, and can take on many forms.

Connective tissues matrix can range from being like liquid, as in the case of blood, to being like sand, as in the case of bone. It is difficult for some people to conceptualize that blood and bone are considered the same types of tissue, but that is the case. Matrix is what gives the connective tissue its different forms such as liquid, rigid, or plastic.

- The form or shape of connective tissue varies greatly. As bone, it can be long and thin, or flat like a cheekbone (the zygomatic process). As fat or part of the skin, it assumes the shape of the underlying tissues it surrounds. Muscle and nervous connective tissues assume a variety of shapes depending on their functions.

- The function of connective tissue is essentially to bind body parts together and to aid the body in functioning. Connective tissues bind and separate body structures (e.g., ligaments and tendons bind, cartilage and facial tissue separate), store and transport nutrients and oxygen (e.g., fatty tissue stores nutrients, blood and lymph tissues transport them), and insulate against heat loss (fatty connective tissue).We can further describe connective tissue by differentiating it into four different types: loose, dense, skeletal, and fluid connective tissues.

3. *Muscle*

- The major identifying characteristic of muscle tissue is its ability to shorten or contract in response to a stimulus. Three types of muscle tissue can be distinguished by the arrangement of their fibers and by the degree to which they may be contracted voluntarily. The three types of muscle tissue are smooth, cardiac, and skeletal.

4. *Nervous*

- Nervous tissue is found throughout the body and is distinguished from other tissues by its excitability and conductivity. There are two kinds of nervous tissue: neural and glial.

- Neural tissue cells are called neurons. They generate and receive stimuli, and process and transmit responses to the body organs through changes in the chemistry of their plasma membranes. These changes are called action potentials. Neurons may be unipolar, bipolar, or multipolar. An example of nervous tissue in the speech mechanism includes the cranial nerves which are responsible for receiving and sending information to and from the oral, pharyngeal, and facial musculature necessary for the production of speech and for swallowing. Another type of nervous tissue is glial tissue or glia. Several types of glia provide support for neural tissue. Glial cells do not generate action potentials, but they are excitable and have important roles in the propagation of action potentials.

C. **Epithelial Tissue**

1. **Characteristics of Epithelial Tissue**

    a. *Intercellular Structure:* Epithelial tissue has very little intercellular material.

    b. *Cellular Arrangement:* Epithelial cells are arranged in a flat or mosaic pattern and are usually situated over a layer of connective tissue.

2. **Functions of Epithelial Tissue**

    a. *Protective:* Epithelial coverings of the outside of the body (the outer skin or epidermis) prevent drying, protect from abrasion, and inhibit the infiltration of micro-organisms.

    b. *Absorptive:* Epithelial tissues line the intestines, absorbing material from the lumen of the gut for nutrition.

    c. *Secretory:* Epithelial cells secrete mucus in the linings of various parts of the body, such as the respiratory tract and stomach.

    d. *Glandular:* Salivary glands, for example, contain secretory epithelial cells. Serous secretory salivary cells secrete watery saliva to help moisten the oral mucosa and digest food. Mucous secretory cells secrete a clear lubricating substance called mucin.

    e. *Sensory:* The epithelia of the ears, eyes, tongue, and nose (to name a few), contain special cells which respond to certain environmental changes by sending an action potential along the nervous tissues to which they are connected.

3. **Types of Epithelial Tissue**

    a. *Proper Epithelium:* Proper epithelium forms the protective inner and outer coverings of the body. This includes the skin as well as the mucous membranes of the digestive tract and airway. The skin of the outer body is connected with the linings of the digestive and respiratory systems. Another word for this connection is continuous. The tissue looks a little different when you compare the outside and the inside, but it is the same type of tissue.

b. *Mesothelium:* Mesothelium forms the protective sac-like walls of the main body cavities. These membranes include the following: the peritoneum, which lines the abdomen; the pleural membranes, which line the inside of the thorax and cover each lung; and the pericardium, which surrounds the heart.

c. *Endothelium:* Endothelium forms the very smooth linings of the blood and lymph vessels.

4. **Descriptive Terms of Epithelial Tissue**

a. **Cell Shape**

One way in which epithelial tissues are described is in terms of the shapes of the composite cells. The shape of an epithelial cell depends, in part, on the mechanical forces acting upon the cell, and in part, on the functions of the cells. A cytoskeleton also provides structure for cell shape.

(1) *Squamous:* Squamous epithelial cells have a flat cell shape. These cells form the inner and outer tissues of parts of the respiratory and digestive tracts and are arranged like the tiles on a floor. Because they are flat, substances can slide over them easily. Squamous cell carcinoma is particularly dangerous, and speech-language pathologists who treat patients who have had their larynges removed surgically (laryngectomy) are aware of the devastating results of such cancer.

(2) *Columnar:* Columnar epithelial cells are cylindrical (long and narrow) and have a functional end. Columnar cells often have little hairs (cilia) at their functional end. One example of a columnar cell is found in the basilar membrane of the cochlea. These hair cells turn acoustic energy into auditory impulses that are sent to the brain to be interpreted as sound. Other examples are found in the nose.

These columnar epithelial cells are activated by chemical changes in the air and are interpreted as smell. Other columnar epithelial cells line the inside of the respiratory tract. They have cilia that wave steadily and help remove debris from the respiratory passages.

    (3)   *Pyramidal:* Pyramidal cells are shaped like pyramids. They are found in the central nervous system. These cells form the pyramidal tracts.

    (4)   *Cuboidal:* Cuboidal cells are shaped like cubes because of the way they are packed in together. These cells can have secretory or absorptive functions.

  b.   **Layers**

    (1)   *Simple:* If there is only one layer, the epithelium is simple. The simple layer can be squamous, columnar, or cuboidal. An example of simple epithelium is in the walls of arteries.

    (2)   *Stratified:* Stratified epithelium is composed of several layers of cells. These layers exist because the tissues are located in places where the outer call layer is exposed to wear. As the outer cells wear off, the lower cells take their places. These cells can be squamous, columnar, or transitional, but the shape description only applies to the outer layer. The surface of the tongue is composed of stratified squamous epithelium.

D.   **Connective Tissue**

  1.   **Characteristics of Connective Tissue**

    Connective tissue has few cells and a large amount of intercellular material (matrix).

    a.   *Variability of Intercellular Structure:* Connective tissue is categorized according to the nature of its matrix. The nonliving matrix is what makes the connective tissue either rigid or plastic.

    b.   *Variability of Form:* Connective tissue can take on various shapes. As bone, it can be long and thin, round or flat. As fat or skin, it can assume the shapes of the underlying tissues it surrounds. Muscle and nervous tissues assume various shapes according to their functions. Another characteristic of connective tissue is that it appears to be able to transmute into other forms. This occurs in the healing process.

2. **Functions of Connective Tissue**

   a. *Structural Binding:* Tendons connect muscles to bones and cartilages; ligaments connect bones to bones, cartilages to cartilages, and cartilages to bones.

   b. *Structural Separation:* Cartilages and fascial tissue separate body structures so they may function relatively freely (without binding against other structures).

   c. *Fatty Connective Tissue Functions:* Store nutrients and insulate against heat loss.

   d. *Fluid Connective Tissue Functions:* Blood has the following functions: oxygenation; evacuation of CO_2 and metabolic waste; nutrition; coagulation; heat distribution; chemical regulation; defense against germs and toxins. Lymph has the following functions: lubrication; anti-infection; transportation of vitamins to the blood to help with the body's immunity.

3. **Types of Connective Tissue**

   a. *Loose Connective Tissue*

   Loose connective tissue forms a base layer to help bind other cell types together and to perform certain functions associated with fat storage. As its name suggests, loose connective tissue matrix fibers are loosely arranged among the ground substance. There are three types of loose connective tissue: areolar, adipose, and reticular.

   (1) *Areolar Tissue:* Areolar connective tissue is a binding type of connective tissue, and it is found all over the body. The connective tissue lying just beneath the skin is areolar connective tissue.

   (2) *Adipose Tissue:* Adipose tissue has special cells that can store fats and oils (triglycerides).

3. *Reticular Tissue:* Reticular tissue is loosely constructed, and, like areolar tissue, serves a binding function in some organs.

b. **Dense Connective Tissue**

Because of its tightly packed fibers and flexible matrix, dense connective tissue is very strong and elastic. Dense connective tissue forms the tendons and ligaments of the body.

(1) *Tendons:* Tendons bind muscles to bones and muscles to muscles. They are very thick and strong, and their fibers are parallel.

(2) *Ligaments:* Ligaments bind bones together and support viscera.

(3) *Aponeuroses:* Aponeuroses are broad flat tendons.

(4) *Fascia:* Fascia are thin sheets of connective tissue that separate bodily structures: muscle bellies separate viscera.

c. **Skeletal Connective Tissue**

(1) **Cartilage**

Cartilage is a flexible skeletal tissue. It gives structure to organs of the respiratory tract and the auditory system and provides cushioning between bones. There are several types of cartilage.

(a) *Hyaline:* Hyaline cartilage is bluish-white and translucent. It forms the skeleton of the larynx and the trachea. With age, this relatively flexible cartilage becomes more rigid in a process called calcification or ossification.

(b) *Elastic:* Elastic cartilage is yellowish and like rubber. It is found in structures that have roles in the production or reception of sound such as the ear canal, some of the smaller cartilages of the larynx, the epiglottis, and the eustachian tubes.

(c)   *Fibrous:* Fibrous cartilage is very tough and immovable. It serves to cushion against shocks and is most notably found within the intervertebral disks of the spine.

2.   **Bone**

Bone, the other type of skeletal connective tissue, is the most rigid connective tissue. It has more intercellular substance than any other tissue type. This intercellular substance, or matrix, is composed of a collagenous substance and ground salts. Ground salts are mostly (~85%) calcium phosphate. Bone cells are sparsely distributed within the matrix and are called osteocytes and osteoblasts. There is a rich system of blood vessels and canals within bone tissue which allows bone to develop fast and heal readily. Bones come in a wide variety of shapes and are classified according to their shapes. The various types of bones include long bones, short bones, flat bones, and irregular bones.

(a)   *Long Bone:* Long bones are longer than they are wide. They form the skeletons of the extremities. There are several parts of a long bone. The shaft forms the long body of the bone. Either end of a long bone is called its ephysis or its head. The smooth surface where bones connect is called an articular facet or condyle.

(b)   *Short Bone:* Short bones in the human body are cube-like and have dimensions that are approximately equal. They include the carpal bones (hands, wrist) and tarsal bones (feet, ankles).

(c)   *Flat Bone:* Flat bones consist of a layer of spongy bone (marrow or diploe) between two thin layers of compact bone. Their cross-section is flat, not rounded. Examples include the skull and ribs. They form the bones of the upper skull (calvaria) and ribs. Flat bones have marrow, but not a bone marrow cavity.

(d)   *Irregular Bone:* Irregular bones have no clear classification, as they have no consistent shape. An obvious example is a vertebra.

(3)   **Articulations of the Skeletal System**

Articulation as a noun refers to the functional union between parts of the body. As a verb it means movement of one part of the body with respect to another. There are several types of articulations. These are classified in two main ways: functional, the degree of movement inherent in the joint; and anatomic, the structures found in the interface of the joints.

(a)   *Functional Classification of Joints*

i)   *Synarthrodial:* Synarthroidal joints are immovable and are found in the sutures of the skull.

ii)   *Amphiarthrodial:* Amphiarthroidal joints are slightly movable and are found in the vertebrae of the spine.

iii)   *Diarthrodial:* Diarthroidal joints are freely movable and are found in the joints of the extremities, the temporo-mandibular, and the cricothyroid joints.

(b)   *Anatomic Classification of Joints*

i)   *Fibrous:* Fibrous joints are like synarthrodial joints having no appreciable movement. The skull sutures are fibrous joints.

ii)   *Cartilaginous:* Cartilaginous joints are like amphiarthroidial joints having little movement. The vertabrae are cartilaginous joints.

iii)   *Synovial:* Synovial joints are freely movable; like diathroidial joints.

(4) **Divisions of the Skeletal System**

(a) *Axial Skeleton:* The axial skeleton is composed of structures associated with the spinal column (axis). Some speech structures associated with the axial skeleton include the ribs, the hyoid bone, the skull, and so forth.

(b) *Appendicular Skeleton:* The appendicular skeleton is formed by structures associated with the upper and lower extremities. These structures attach to the axial skeleton.

4. **Fluid Connective Tissue**

Fluid connective tissue forms the blood and lymph. This type of connective tissue is distinct in terms of the loose nature of the molecular bonds of its intercellular matrix.

a. *Blood*

- Blood is a very specialized form of connective tissue. It consists of red blood cells, white blood cells, platelets, and a yellowish transparent fluid called "plasma." Blood has several functions which are listed below. Related to the speech mechanism, blood is responsible for transporting oxygen and carbon dioxide to and from the cells, an important component of respiration.

- *Oxygenation, Nutrition, Evacuation:* Blood transports oxygen and carbon dioxide to and from the cells; transports nutrients to the cells and waste material from them; transports hormones to the cells.

- *Heat Distribution and Chemical Regulation:* Blood regulates body temperature; regulates acid/alkali balance (pH); and regulates water composition of the cells.

- *Healing:* Blood coagulates to prevent blood loss following injury.

- *Immunity:* Blood defends against destructive microorganisms and destroys certain poisons.

b. *Lymph*

Lymph, the other type of fluid connective tissue, functions to transport lipids and vitamins to the blood and to fight infection.

E.   **Muscle Tissue**

1.   **Characteristics of Muscle Tissue**

The major identifying characteristic of muscle tissue is its contractile property. Contractibility refers to the ability to shorten. It is important to remember that muscles can only shorten. They must rely on another muscle to pull them back to an elongated position.

2.   **Functions of Muscle Tissue**

a.   *Sarcomere:* A sarcomere is the smallest contractile unit in the muscle contractile hierarchy. Muscle contraction starts at the molecular level. The molecules are so small we can only see them with a powerful electron microscope. They are only components of the first and smallest contractile unit. The molecules actin and myosin slide together when their electrochemical properties are changed by the nervous system. Sarcomeres are bundles of these molecules. As the actin and myosin slide together they become more compact and shorten, creating the sarcomere. The muscle is built up of successively larger components, each shortening because the next smaller component is getting shorter.

b.   *Myofibril:* A myofibril is a collection of sarcomeres laid end-to-end. It is easy to imagine that when the sarcomeres get shorter the myofibril will also get shorter.

c.   *Muscle Fiber:* The next largest contractile unit is the muscle fiber. A muscle fiber is also called a muscle cell because it is the basic structural unit of muscle tissue. Muscle cells have sarcomeres as part of their cytostructure. These specialized cells may have more than one nucleus.

d.   *Muscle Fasciculus:* A muscle fasciculus is a group of muscle cells and is our next largest muscle contractile unit. A fasciculus is a group of muscle fibers.

e.   *Muscle:* The largest contractile unit in the hierarchy is simply a muscle. Muscles have identifying names and these names may refer to their locations, shapes, or functions.

3. **Types of Muscle Tissue**

    There are three types of muscle tissue: smooth, cardiac, and skeletal. These types of muscle tissue can be distinguished by the arrangements of their fibers and by the degree to which they may be contracted voluntarily.

    a. *Smooth:* Smooth muscle tissue is also called visceral muscle tissue. It forms the muscles of the internal organs and blood vessels. Smooth muscle tissue is controlled by involuntary (autonomic) nervous action. It controls internal functions, such as digestion and glandular secretion. An exception to this is the branchial musculature at the anterior end of the alimentary (digestive) tract. These muscles are under voluntary control, and are not smooth muscles. Instead, they are striated or skeletal muscles. They include, of course, the muscles of the speech system.

    b. *Cardiac:* Cardiac muscle tissue is only found in the heart. It has certain characteristics of the other two muscle types.

    c. *Striated:* Striated or skeletal muscle tissue is under voluntary control. This means we can contract skeletal muscles when we want to or let them relax when not needed. This kind of muscle tissue is characterized by parallel fibers.

4. **Muscle Feedback**

    Conscious muscle feedback takes the form of touch sensations generated by special organs in the muscles as they move or as they stop moving. These sensations allow the speaker to be aware of the movement and position of the articulators in order to correct them as necessary. Not all muscle feedback is conscious. Some feedback reaches the central nervous system at unconscious levels for much faster regulation than would be possible if a conscious decision were required.

5. **Muscle Attachment**

    a. *Origin:* The origin of a muscle is the end attached to the relatively fixed part; the part that does not move.

    b. *Insertion:* The insertion of a muscle is the end attached to the relatively movable part. Some muscles are named in terms of their origins and insertions. In those cases, the name is the origin first, then the insertion.

6. **Muscle Function Terminology**

a. *Flexion:* Bringing of appendicular or axial structures into closer proximity; curling up.

b. *Extension:* Stretching structures to their greatest length.

c. *Adduction:* Bringing structures toward the midline.

d. *Abduction:* Moving structures away from midline.

7. **Names of Muscles**

a. *Shape:* Some muscles are named according to their visual characteristics. An example is the digastric muscle found in the neck. Digastric means "two bellies."

b. *Function:* Some are named in Latin for their action. An example is levator labii superiorus: lifter of the upper lip.

c. *Location:* Some are named for where they are found. An example is the mentalis: located at the mental eminence. The mental eminence is at the tip of the chin.

F. **Nervous Tissue**

1. **Characteristics of Nervous Tissue**

a. *Excitability:* Excitability is the capacity to respond to some type of triggering event. These events are called stimuli (a single event is called a stimulus). Stimuli can be physical in the form of mechanical movement or pressure (a poke), or in the form of light, heat, or sound. Stimuli can also be chemical in the form of molecules in the atmosphere, on the tongue or in the inner body. All that is needed is a special kind of organ (often composed of epithelial tissue) to convert the stimulus into a chemical change. Nervous tissue cells, called neurons, have special mechanisms that make them extremely susceptible to changes in the chemistry on their cell membranes. These cell membranes are chemically balanced, like a battery that is not connected to anything. A stimulus upsets this balance and causes a special chain reaction that enables the neuron to function.

b.   *Conductivity:* Conductivity refers to the special property of nervous tissue to channel its excitement in a certain direction. Due to the chemical balance of the cell membrane, the excitement travels in one direction along only the surface of the neuron. When there is no excitement on the cell membrane the neuron is at rest or polarized. This means the chemical electric charge on the inside and outside of the membrane is balanced. However, it does not take much to tip the balance and "start the show." The upset of chemical balance, or depolarization, along the neuron cell membrane is called an action potential. It is the action potential that makes neurons function. Action potentials can be started by any stimulus including the effects of another neuron. Action potential depolarization moves along the membranes of the neurons. When one location on the membrane is depolarized it affects the location next to it on the membrane. As soon as that happens the first location tends to return to its normal resting state. Action potential depolarization is said to be propagated in this manner, with one location on the cell membrane becoming depolarized and returning to normal, while an adjacent location becomes depolarized and the wave moves on.

2.   **Functions of Nervous Tissue**

a.   *Excitatory:* Excitatory functions are those which cause the neuron to act.

b.   *Inhibitory:* Inhibitory functions are those which keep the neuron from acting when action is not desirable.

3.   **Types of Nervous Tissue**

a.   *Neurons*

(1)   *Unipolar Neurons:* True unipolar neurons are rare in the nervous system. They are most often seen in developing embryos and fetuses and eventually grow into one of the other types. Unipolar neurons have a single process attached to a cell body. This single process extends a short distance from the cell body and then splits into two sections. One of the sections acts as a dendrite and conducts action potentials toward the cell body while the other acts as an axon. Pseudounipolar neurons

are bipolar neurons that have changed to appear like unipolar neurons. They are found in the brain and spinal cord and are best known for conveying action potentials associated with the sense of touch from the extremities to the brain and spinal cord.

(2)   ***Bipolar Neurons:*** Bipolar neurons have a cell body and two projections opposite one another. One is afferent and the other is efferent. Bipolar neurons are usually found in the organs of the special senses: vision, hearing, smell, balance, and taste.

(3)   ***Multipolar Neurons:*** The most common types of neurons are multipolar neurons. These come in many shapes, but basically consist of a cell body with more than two projections extending away. Some look like Koosh balls whereas others look like little pyramids with long axons and many dendrites. They are all found in the brain and spinal cord. The best known multipolar neurons are those that conduct action potentials associated with voluntary movement of the muscles from the brain to the spinal cord.

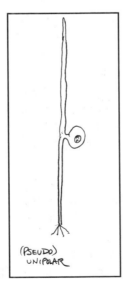
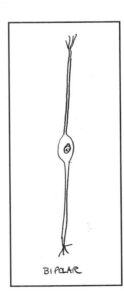
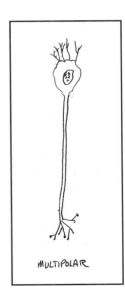

b.   ***Neuroglial Cells:*** In the central nervous system, neurons are embedded in a special connective tissue matrix called neuroglia. These neuroglia cells support, insulate, and nourish the neurons.

(1) *Myelinating Glia (Oligodendrocytes):* These cells have smaller cell bodies (than even the astrocytes) and very few processes. They grow in a spiral around the axons of neurons and appear to have several functions. They serve a nutritive and protective function, provide insulation between adjacent neurons, and play a role in deposition and maintenance of the myelin sheath.

(2) *Astrocytes:* Astrocytes are star-shaped (stellate) cells that almost completely surround the neurons. They have small cell bodies and elaborate branching processes. Astrocytes' processes project to the synapses between neurons and react to the presence of chemical substances generated therein. Astrocytes give support to the neurons. Some anatomists feel that they serve an intermediary function between the capillaries and the neurons in the supply of nutrition. The two types of astrocytes are protoplasmic and fibrous. Following a lesion or degeneration of the CNS, astrocytes proliferate to a hyperplastic state.

(3) *Microglia:* Microglia cells are very amoeboid (flexible) and phagocytic. They exist in the interstices of the dense CNS tissue. They are mesodermal (not ectodermal) in origin. When microglia are exposed to inflammatory conditions, they undergo changes. Their processes withdraw into the swollen cell body, and each assumes a round form. Microglia play an important role in the removal and ingestion of degenerative debris or blood clots following hemorrhage.

(4) *Neurilemma (Ependymal Cells):* These cells form the lining of the neural tube, including the cerebral ventricles. This lining prevents the fluid of the ventricles and spinal canal from entering the brain tissue. Neurilemmas also secrete and absorb cerebrospinal fluid (CSF. and help CSF circulate.

G. **Tissue Differentiation**

1. **Germ Layers**

Germ layers form during the earliest developmental changes that occur in the human body. Cells which were, at first, all identical (or nearly so) in form and function begin to develop different characteristics. These changes take place while the individual is still in the womb (uterus) being formed. During this prenatal stage, the individual is referred to as an embryo. About nine weeks after conception, the individual is called a fetus. In a fetus differentiated body systems begin to appear and develop.

a.   *Endoderm:* The internal organs develop from the endoderm.

b.   *Mesoderm:* Muscles, connective tissue, and deep skin develop from the mesoderm.

c.   *Ectoderm:* From the ectoderm develops the outer layer of skin, the linings of the oral and nasal cavities, and the nervous system.

2.   **Branchial Arches**

The branchial arches are the six pieces of cartilage or bone in the anterior end of the alimentary canal. Each arch includes the cartilaginous arch, a nerve, an artery and a vein.

a.   **First Arch (Mandibular Arch)**

(1)   **Maxillary Section**

(a)   **Superior Oral Cavity (anterior 2/3)**

(b)   **Superior Lip**

(c)   **Incus**

(d)   **Maxillary Division of Trigeminal Nerve**

(2)   **Mandibular Section**

(a)   **Mandible**

(b)   **Anterior Two-Thirds of Tongue**

(c)   **Inferior Lip**

(d)   **Muscles of Mastication**

(e)   **Malleus**

(f)   **Mandibular Division of Trigeminal Nerve**

b. Second Arch (Hyoid Arch)

(1) Stapes

(2) Upper Body and Lesser Cornua of Hyoid

(3) Muscles of Facial Expression

(4) Facial Nerve

c. Third Arch

(1) Lower Body and Greater Horns of Hyoid

(2) Posterior One-Third of Tongue

(3) Stylopharyngeus Muscle

(4) Glossopharyngeal Nerve

d. Fourth Arch

(1) Epiglottis

(2) Thyroid Cartilage

(3) Cuneiform Cartilages

(4) Pharyngeal Constrictors and Cricothyroid Muscle

(5) Superior Laryngeal Nerve

e. Fifth Arch

(1) (Obliterated Early in Development)

f. Sixth Arch

(1) Intrinsic Laryngeal Muscles except for the Crico-thyroid muscle.

(2) Recurrent Laryngeal Nerve

IV.   **Organs and Systems**

   A.   **Definitions**

      1.   *System:* A system is a group of organs that perform a specific function. There are at least nine systems in the body that all interact to produce life sustaining action. Several interact to produce acts of communication.

      2.   *Organ:* An organ is a collection of tissues that perform a specific function.

   B.   **Review of Systems and Their Interactions**

      1.   *Respiratory:* The respiratory system is required to produce a column of air upon which to superimpose speech. Normal speech requires air from the lungs. The primary function of the respiratory system is not for speech. It provides gases for metabolism. Without these gases, the organism would die.

      2.   *Nervous:* The function of the nervous system is to convey stimuli to and from the brain.

      3.   *Muscular:* The function of the muscular system is to enable movement.

      4.   *Circulatory:* The circulatory, digestive, urinary, endocrine, and vascular systems all play a role in keeping the body functioning.

      5.   *Digestive:* The circulatory, digestive, urinary, endocrine, and vascular systems all play a role in keeping the body functioning.

      6.   *Urinary:* The circulatory, digestive, urinary, endocrine, and vascular systems all play a role in keeping the body functioning.

      7.   *Endocrine:* The circulatory, digestive, urinary, endocrine, and vascular systems all play a role in keeping the body functioning.

      8.   *Vascular:* The circulatory, digestive, urinary, endocrine, and vascular systems all play a role in keeping the body functioning.

      9.   *Skeletal:* The skeletal, integumentary, and articular systems provide the structure of the body so physical signals can be produced.

10. *Integumentary:* The skeletal, integumentary, and articular systems provide the structure of the body so physical signals can be produced.

11. *Articular:* The skeletal, integumentary, and articular systems provide the structure of the body so physical signals can be produced.

UNIT 3

THE RESPIRATORY MECHANISM

I. **Two Definitions for Respiration**

- The primary function of the respiratory system is to provide the exchange of gases necessary for cell metabolism, a process essential for life itself. This primary function takes precedence over all secondary respiratory functions. The same process by which gas moves in and out of the respiratory system also provides the pressure necessary to drive the speech mechanism.

- The speech function of the respiratory system makes it obvious why speech-language pathologists need to understand this dynamic system. However speech-language pathologists also work with individuals who have difficulty swallowing (dysphagia). In addition to the importance of respiration for speech, swallowing disorders that result in aspiration (entry of a foreign substance into the lungs) cause problems with breathing. For both of these reasons, speech-language pathologists find knowledge of the respiratory system a necessity. Often, therapy may focus specifically on improving respiration and other times the focus may be only on a component of the system.

- The two main functions of the respiratory system are to maintain cell metabolism and to provide a column of compressed air for speech. Of these two, by far the most important is the first, the biological function.

A. **Physical**

The physical definition of respiration is: the process of gas exchange between an organism and its environment. There are three phases of physical respiration: pulmonary ventilation (breathing); external (pulmonary) respiration; and internal (tissue) respiration.

1. **Biological Functions**

- The biological function of the respiratory system is to provide a means of gas exchange between the human being and the environment. This means bringing in oxygen to the cells and carrying away carbon dioxide. The air we inhale contains about 20% oxygen, and the air we exhale contains about 16% oxygen. The oxygen that is missing from the air we exhale (breathe out) was used by the cells.

- Although not quite as important, there are some other biological functions of the respiratory system. These include bringing gases to the olfactory (smell) end organs to provide the sense of the chemical content of the air around us, as well as to filter and moisturize the air we inhale.

2. **Speech Function**

The respiratory system also provides a column of compressed air for the production of speech. With this air we can produce sounds by forcing it through closed or nearly closed structures of the vocal tract. There are three basic kinds of sounds we make with this compressed air. First, we use it to drive the vocal folds open and closed in rapid succession. This produces the sound of the voice: phonation. Phonation is heard when we produce vowel sounds and voiced consonants (e.g., /b/, /v/, /g/, /n/).We also may trap the air, let pressure build up, and then suddenly release it. This produces a popping sound we call a plosive (e.g., /p/ and /b/ and /t/ and /d/). Finally, we may choose to force the air through a tight constriction. This makes a hissing sound we call a "fricative" (e.g., /ʃ/, /f/, /v/, and, /s/).

B. **Chemical**

The chemical or cellular definition of respiration describes the process of metabolism. Metabolism is the process by which cells create energy. The process is quite complicated, but put simply, involves converting sugar (or hydrocarbons) and oxygen into carbon dioxide and water. This process creates energy and keeps the cells functioning. A chemist would write the metabolism equation this way: $C_6H_{12}O_6 + 6O_2 \rightarrow 6CO_2 + 6H_2O$

II. **Structures of the Respiratory Tract**

A. **Location of the Respiratory System**

- Respiratory structures are located in the chest (thoracic region) and in the head and neck (cranial and cervical regions). The thoracic area, encompassing the lungs and trachea, is the lower respiratory tract. The cervical region, encompassing the nasal, oral, and pharyngeal regions is considered the upper respiratory tract, or vocal tract.

- The respiratory system consists of the respiratory passages and the lungs. The respiratory passages are tubes that connect the lungs to the outside environment allowing gases to flow into and out of the lungs. In that sense, they are just like the ducts that let air flow through your home or car heating system, except these ducts are living tissues. The respiratory passages include (from outside to inside) the nasal passages (nasal cavity), nasal pharynx, oral cavity (mouth), oral pharynx, larynx, trachea, and bronchial tree. Most of the bronchial tree is embedded in the substance of the lung. The lungs are the organs where gas exchange occurs. There are two lungs, located on either side of the thoracic cavity. Inside each lung are tiny spaces where the bloodstream receives and emits gases from and to the respiratory passages. This gas exchange is necessary for cell metabolism.

1.   **Upper Respiratory Tract**

The upper respiratory tract extends from the inferior border of the larynx to the openings of the nose (the nares or nostrils).

2.   **Lower Respiratory Tract**

The lower respiratory tract extends from the lungs to the inferior end of the larynx (superior end of the trachea).

B.   **Skeleton of the Respiratory Tract**

The skeleton of the respiratory tract is composed of the spinal column, pelvic girdle, rib cage, clavicles, scapulae, and skull. These bones protect the soft tissues of the respiratory system and provide attachments for the muscles that power it. They form the axial skeleton of the human body.

1.   **Spinal Column**

The spinal column is a series of irregular bones extending from the base of the skull to the pelvis. It houses the spinal cord in the intervertebral canal. It is fairly common to confuse the spinal column with the spinal cord. The column is a stack of bones, and the cord is a collection of soft nerve tissue.

a.   **Vertebrae**

The bones of the spinal column are called vertebrae. One of these bones is called a vertebra. Typically, there are 33 vertebrae divided into 5 distinct types, depending on where in the body the vertebrae are located. The actual number varies from person to person, but there are usually 7 cervical, 12 thoracic, 5 lumbar, 5 sacral, and 4 coccygeal vertebrae. The sacral and coccygeal vertebrae are fused.

(1)   **Structure**

Each vertebra has a thick body, which articulates with the vertebrae above and below it, and bears the weight of the anatomy superior to it. You will notice that vertebrae are relatively small at the superior end of the column and become progressively larger inferiorly. The larger size of the inferior vertebrae enables them to bear the greater weight imposed by the superior body parts. Posterior to the body of each vertebra is a vertebral arch. The arches and bodies of each vertebra form a vertebral foramen; when stacked they form the vertebral canal. The vertebral canal contains the spinal cord, membranes, and the roots of the spinal nerves. Vertebrae also have two processes extending laterally. These are called transverse processes and serve as attachments for muscles of the spine. Another process of each vertebra extends posteriorly. This is called the spinous process.

(2) **Types of Vertebrae**

(a) ***Cervical:*** In the cervical region there are seven vertebrae. They are distinguished by the foramina (holes) in their transverse processes. The vertebral arteries pass through these stacked foramina on their way to the brain.

    i) **Special Names for Cervebrae:** Three cervical vertebrae have special names, in addition to their C-names.

(b) ***Atlas:*** C-1, the first cervical vertebra is called atlas. The atlas, which holds up the head, was named after the mythical Greek character who supposedly holds up the Earth.

(c) ***Axis:*** The second cervical vertebra, C-2, is called axis because most rotation of the skull in relationship to the neck occurs at the joint between axis and atlas. This is called the atlantoaxial joint.

(d) ***Vertebra Prominens:*** C-7 is called vertebra prominens because its spinous process is easily felt (palpated) beneath the skin.

(e) ***Thoracic:*** There are 12 thoracic vertebrae distinguished by their articular facets for the twelve ribs. Ribs articulate with thoracic vertebrae at the costovertebral joints.

(f) ***Lumbar:*** The five lumbar vertebrae are distinguished by their lack of transverse process foramina, lack of costal articular facets, and by their great size. The great size of the lumbar vertebrae enables them to bear the weight of the superior anatomy.

(g)   *Sacral:* The five sacral vertebrae form the pelvic girdle along with two hip bones. This part of the body made up of sacral vertebrae is called the sacrum.

(h)   *Coccygeal:* Three or four coccygeal vertebrae form the coccyx. These are fused to the pelvic bones.

2.   **Pelvic Girdle**

The pelvic girdle provides attachments for the muscles of the abdominal wall which function in breathing. It also forms a floor for the abdominal viscera against which the diaphragm, the primary muscle of inspiration, pushes during breathing.

3.   **Rib Cage**

a.   *Ribs:* Twelve paired ribs and the sternum form a protective cage around the heart and lungs. The ribs are flexible and articulate with the vertebrae and sternum with a cartilaginous joint. Only the first 10 ribs articulate with the sternum anteriorly. The last two have no anterior articulation. These are called floating ribs.

b.   *Sternum:* The sternum is also called the breastbone. It forms a rigid shield in the center of the thorax. Ribs 1 to 10 attach anteriorly to the sternum. The attachment is called the sternocostal ligament.

4.   **Clavicles**

The clavicles are also called the collar bones. These serve as attachments for the accessory muscles of respiration. The clavicle is the most commonly broken bone in the body because of the natural tendency for a person to extend the arms during a forward fall. The impact of the fall is often transmitted through the bones of the upper extremity to the clavicle.

5.   **Scapulae**

The scapulae are often called the shoulder bones. The scapulae also serve as attachments for accessory muscles of respiration.

C.   **Nose and Nasal Cavity**

1.   ***Nares:*** The nares are located at the distal tip of the nose and form the entrance to the nasal cavity. These prominent facial landmarks are also called the nostrils.

2.   ***Septum:*** Between the two nares, choanae, and the passages to which they give entrance is the nasal septum. The nasal septum is a wall separating the nasal passages. It is formed of cartilage and bone. The bones of the nasal septum include the ethmoid bone and the vomer. The cartilages of the nasal septum are the septal cartilage and the greater alar cartilage.

3.   ***Root:*** The root of the nose is the point at which the nasal bones articulate with the face. Here the bones include the maxillae and the frontal bone.

4.   ***Choanae:*** The choanae are the posterior openings of the nasal passages. The choanae open into the upper part of the pharynx, called the nasopharynx.

D.   **Pharynx**

The part of the respiratory passage that connects the trachea with the oral and nasal cavities is of particular interest to speech-language pathologists. This passage is called the pharynx, and it has three divisions.

1.   ***Nasopharynx:*** The most superior division of the pharynx is located posterior to the nasal cavity, or nose. Because it connects the nasal cavity (passages) to the respiratory passages, the superior part of the pharynx is called the nasopharynx.

2.   ***Oropharynx:*** The middle portion of the pharynx is located right behind the oral cavity. Because it connects the oral cavity to the respiratory passages, the middle division of the pharynx is called the oropharynx.

3.   ***Laryngopharynx:*** The most inferior part of the pharynx connects it to the trachea. It also contains the larynx, a series of muscular valves that protect the airway entrance and produce the voice. Because it contains the larynx, the inferior division of the pharynx is called the laryngopharynx.

E.   **Oral Cavity Structure and Function**

   1.   ***Fauces:*** At the posterior end of the oral cavity, as mentioned above, are the fauces or faucial arches. You can see these arches toward the back of the mouth when looking in a mirror. They are also called the oropharyngeal isthmus. There is an anterior faucial arch and a posterior faucial arch on each side of the oral cavity.

   2.   ***Triangular Fossa***: The space between the two fauces is called the triangular fossa. A fossa is a depressed area. There is a triangular fossa on either side of the posterior oral cavity.

   3.   ***Tonsils:*** The tonsils are three masses of lymphoid tissue in the oropharynx and in the oral cavity. These protect the airway from bacterial invasions. In the triangular fossa (between the faucial arches) lie the palatine tonsils, one on either side. At the posterior part of the tongue is the lingual tonsil. Up in the pharynx, where the oropharynx and nasopharynx meet, is the pharyngeal tonsil also called the adenoid. The pharyngeal, palatine, and lingual tonsils form Waldeyer's ring encircling the nasal and oral portions of the pharynx.

F.   **Laryngopharynx**

   The laryngopharynx extends from the laryngeal inlet to the first tracheal ring. It lies behind and partially around the larynx, which is its principal structure. Like many of the other respiratory tract structures, the larynx has a biological and a speech function. The biological function is to protect the airway from the intrusion of foreign objects. The speech function is to provide a phonatory source for speech.

G.   **Trachea**

   •   The trachea, or windpipe, extends down from the inferior border of the larynx to the level of the fifth thoracic vertebra. It consists of 15 to 20 cartilaginous rings and is incomplete posteriorly. The trachea is held together by connective tissue and muscle. The cartilaginous rings help it maintain its patency (openness), so air can freely flow to and from the lungs.

   •   The trachea lies anterior to the esophagus for its entire course. The esophagus is located between the spine and the trachea. The trachea is flexible, and in this respect is similar to a vacuum cleaner hose. It needs to be flexible because it moves about freely during breathing, swallowing, and with changes in body posture.

H.   Bronchial Tree

1.   *Main Stem Bronchi:* At the level of the fifth thoracic vertebra the trachea splits to form the twin main stem bronchi. There is one bronchus for each lung. These respiratory passages are also known as bronchial tubes. The bronchi are not identical. The one on the right is straighter as it enters the right lung, while the one on the left takes a lateral course to provide space for the heart. Aspirated substances are more likely to enter the right lung because of the straight passage of the right tube. The bronchial tubes enter each lung, but there is a short part of each one that remains outside the substance of the lung. This part is called extrapulmonary. Once the bronchi enter the lung, they are said to be intrapulmonary. Inside the lungs the bronchial tubes branch out into smaller but more numerous branches of the bronchial tree.

2.   *Secondary Bronchi:* The next divisions of the bronchial tree are the secondary, or lobar, bronchi.

3.   *Tertiary Bronchi:* Secondary bronchi are followed by the tertiary bronchi.

4.   *Bronchioles:* The smallest branches of the bronchial tree are bronchioles or terminal bronchi.

I.   Lungs

1.   *Right and Left Lung Differences:* There are two lungs: a right lung and a left lung. The right lung has three lobes: upper, middle, and lower. The left lung has two lobes: upper and lower. Remember that the heart is located near the medial surface of the left lung.

2.   *Alveoli:* Tiny sacks called alveoli line the walls of the terminal bronchi. It is here that the exchange of gas takes place. The exchange is enhanced by the extremely thin surface membrane and large area of contact between the blood inside the alveoli and the air inside the bronchi.

3.   *Pleurae:* Each lung is surrounded by two pleural membranes, the visceral and parietal pleurae. Between the membranes is a fluid called intrapleural fluid. The pleural membranes are held together in part by the surface tension of this fluid in much the same way a saucer becomes stuck to the bottom of a coffee cup when some of the coffee is spilled in the saucer.

a.   *Intrapleural Fluid:* The intrapleural fluid is the fluid between the visceral and parietal pleura that keeps these two membranes together.

b.   *Visceral Pleura:* Each lung is covered with a layer of visceral pleura.

c.   *Parietal Pleura:* Each lung and its visceral pleura are contained in a sack of parietal pleura. The parietal pleurae absorb gases to create negative pressure in the space between the pleura (intrapleural space). This forces the pleura to stick together (normally) and resist the tendency of the lungs to retract from the medial surface of the thorax. The lungs can collapse if the attraction between the pleurae is disturbed, causing a pneumothorax.

III.   Mechanics of Respiration

A.   Boyle's Law

- The muscles of the respiratory system act on the skeleton and soft tissues of the respiratory system to allow it to move gases in and out of the lungs and respiratory passages. They do this by changing the dimensions of the thorax. Two physical principles ensure the flow of air in and out of the respiratory system: Boyle's law and the second law of thermodynamics. Boyle's law (Robert Boyle, 1662) states that, "The volume of a fixed amount of gas maintained at a constant temperature is inversely proportional to the pressure of that gas." This means that increasing the volume of a container of gas two-fold will result in its pressure being reduced by one-half (and so on). That is, if you make the container holding a given amount of substance (air) bigger, the pressure of that substance against the interior walls of the container will be less.

- The second law of thermodynamics posits that there is a natural tendency for a substance, such as air, to flow from high pressure environments to low pressure environments until the pressures in both environments are equal. Thus, when we expand our chests (thoraxes) we increase the internal volume of the lungs. This expansion lowers the pressure inside the lungs relative to the atmospheric pressure outside the lungs. The natural tendency is for the air outside, under higher pressure, to flow into the lungs until the two pressures are equal. Conversely, when we let our chests relax, allowing them to shrink back down to their normal resting size and volume, it causes the air pressure inside to become greater than the pressure outside, and the flow is reversed. The gas is forced out of the respiratory system due to the natural tendency for substances under pressure to equalize. The higher pressured gas inside the lungs will flow out to the lower pressure of the environment to equalize pressures. During expiration, the air has less oxygen and more carbon dioxide because of the gas exchange that took place in the lungs.

B.   **Inspiration and Expiration**

    1.   **Respiratory Cycle**

A respiratory cycle consists of one inspiration and one expiration. Inspiration occurs when air flows into the lungs with contraction of the muscles of inspiration. This expands the thorax, creating momentary negative internal pressure causing air to rush in and equalize the pressure. Expiration occurs when air flows out of the system in conjunction with contraction of the thorax. As each phase takes up a portion of the total time of the respiratory cycle, the respiratory cycle can be described in terms of how much time (seconds) it takes to accomplish each phase. The ratio of the duration of inspiration to the total time for the cycle is called the I-Fraction.

       a.   *Vegetative Breathing:* Normal breathing for life maintenance is called vegetative breathing. The I-Fraction for normal vegetative breathing is approximately 0.45 seconds. This means inspiration normally takes a little less than half the time of the whole cycle.

       b.   *Respiration for Speech:* The respiratory cycle for speech differs from that in vegetative breathing. The I-fraction for speech is approximately 0.16. This means that inspiration for speech takes up less than one-fifth (I = 0.16) of the respiratory cycle time. Speech requires quick inspiration and slow expiration.

    2.   **Respiratory Rates**

Respiratory rate refers to the number of respiratory cycles per minute. Respiratory rates are measured by observing the movements of the body during breathing. Inspiration is observed when the dimensions of the thorax or abdomen are increased. To determine respiratory rate, the observer counts the number of inspirations and expirations for 30 seconds. Those figures are then multiplied by 2.

       a.   *Adult Respiratory Rate Range:* 12 to 30 cycles per minute

b. *Child Respiratory Rate Range:*

1 to 5 years: 25 to 40 cycles per minute

5 to 12 years: 12 to 36 cycles per minute

c. *Infant Respiratory Rate Range:* 30 to 70 cycles per minute.

3. **Respiratory Patterns**

a. **Normal Patterns of Respiration**

(1) **Diaphragmatic/Abdominal**

Maximum displacement is in the area below the ribs. There is some thoracic movement, which increases as the individual concentrates on the act of breathing.

(2) **Thoracic**

Maximum displacement is in the thoracic region. This is a normal pattern, but is not as efficient as the diaphragmatic/abdominal pattern.

(3) **Clavicular**

Maximum displacement is in the suprasternal area with pronounced clavicular movement. An inefficient pattern by itself, the clavicular pattern is used by individuals starved for air or limited in function of the respiratory mechanism. Clavicular breathing uses all of the accessory muscles of inspiration.

b. **Pathologic Patterns of Respiration**

(1) **Cheyne-Stokes Respiration**

This pattern consists of rapid, irregular breathing for 30 seconds to 2 minutes. Respiration starts with shallow volumes, gets deeper, then shallow again. Breathing alternates with periods of apnea (no breathing) for 5 to 30 seconds. Cheyne-Stokes respiration results from central nervous system (CNS) dysfunction.

(2) **Neurogenic Hyperventilation**

This pattern is one of deep, rapid respiration. Deep respiration is called hyperpnea; rapid respiration is called tachypnea. Neurogenic hyperventilation can be caused by head trauma or diabetic coma.

(3)   **Kussmaul Respiration**

This pattern is one of deep sighing breathing. It is seen in diabetic ketoacidosis or air hunger.

C.   Muscles of Respiration

1.   Function of the Muscles of Respiration

a.   Diaphragmatic Movement

The most important primary muscle of inspiration is the diaphragm. The diaphragm is an umbrella-shaped muscle located under the lungs. It is the anatomic border between the thoracic and abdominal regions of the body. When the fibers of the diaphragm contract they cause the dome shape of the entire muscle to become flatter. Because the muscle forms the floor of the thoracic cavity, this flattening increases the top-to-bottom volume of the thorax. As the thorax becomes larger the lungs also become larger because the lungs are attracted to the thoracic wall by pleural linkage.

b.   Costal Movement

The diaphragm is not the only primary muscle of inspiration. Several sets of muscles help change thoracic dimensions by acting on the ribs. This type of movement is called costal movement. There are two-dimensional changes in the thorax brought about by costal movement.

(1)   **"Pump Handle"**

Pump-handle movement moves the thorax up and forward. This movement is accomplished by movement of ribs 1 through 6.

(2)   **"Bucket Handle"**

Bucket-handle movement moves up and laterally, by action of ribs 7 through 10.

2.   Inspiration: Active Movement

a.   Primary Muscles of Inspiration

(1)   **Diaphragm**

The diaphragm is a large muscle and has many points of origin. Some of the origins are peripheral and some central, contributing to the diaphragm's flat, domelike shape. Peripherally, muscle fibers originate from the xiphoid process of the sternum, the deep aspects of the lower six costal (rib) cartilages, and the bodies of the first two or three lumbar vertebrae. Central fibers arise from their attachments to the upper three or four lumbar vertebrae to three ligaments on either side of the spine as well as the lateral and medial arcuate ligaments.

(2)   **Intercostal Muscles**

The muscles that make the ribs move forward and up (pump handle movement) and up and lateral (bucket handle movement) are the external intercostal muscles. There are 11 pairs of external intercostal muscles and they are located on each side of the thorax. On each set of ribs these muscles attach to the lateral side of the costal groove (just medial and above the inferior border) of an upper rib, lateral border of first rib, and to the upper border of the rib below.

b.   **Secondary Muscles of Inspiration**

When an individual needs to move air, such as when he or she is under exertion or disease conditions, the secondary (accessory) muscles of inspiration come into play. Secondary muscles of inspiration pull the thoracic walls a little more to move the maximum amount of air. The following muscles are the secondary muscles of inspiration.

(1)   *Pectoralis Majorus/Minoris:* The pectoralis muscles originate at the clavicle, sternum, and cartilage of ribs 1 to 6. They insert on the lateral aspect of the anterior humerus. Pectoralis minor lies just below pectoralis major.

(2)   *Costal Levators:* There are 12 costal elevators on either side of the rib cage. They arise from the transverse processes of the seventh cervical and upper 11 thoracic vertebrae. They insert between the tubercle and the angle of the rib immediately below.

(3)   *Serratus Anteriorus:* These muscles are located between the ribs and the scapulae. They arise from

the side of ribs 1 through 8 or 9 and insert along the vertebral border of the scapulae.

(4) ***Serratus Posterior Superiorus:*** This muscle originates from a broad tendon at the spinous process of the seventh cervical vertebrae and inserts just lateral to the angles on ribs 2 through 5.

(5) ***Latissimus Dorsi:*** The latissimus dorsi arises from the spine of the lower thoracic vertebrae, the lumbar vertebrae, the sacrum, and from the posterior third of the iliac crest by means of a broad aponeurosis. The fibers insert into the upper humerus by means of a stout tendon.

(6) ***Scalenus:*** This muscle originates on the transverse process of the cervical vertebrae and inserts on the two uppermost ribs: C-3 through C-6, to ribs 1 and 2.

3. **Expiration**

   a. **Passive Movement:** Expiration is usually a passive function. During normal expiration the thorax is allowed to contract through its natural elasticity. In other words, action or contraction of the muscles of expiration is minimal or nonexistent during normal breathing. Instead, the muscles of inspiration relax, allowing the thorax to return to its natural resting shape passively. Muscles of expiration are only used when it is necessary to contract the thorax beyond its neutral or relaxed state.

   b. **Active Movement:** In speech the muscles of expiration may be used when emphasis or stress is required or when the speaker is trying to utter a particularly long passage without stopping. Normally the muscles of inspiration are active during speech, gradually relaxing their tonus (contractile state). This allows the thorax to slowly return to the resting state and prolong the flow of air out of the system.

      (1) **Muscles of Expiration:** The primary muscles of expiration are active for mild sustained voluntary expiration. Secondary muscles are active under conditions of stress.

(a)　**Primary Muscles of Expiration**

　i)　*Internal Intercostals:* The internal intercostals originate at the lower borders of the upper 11 ribs. From there they course down to insert onto the medial aspect of the rib immediately below.

　ii)　*Rectus Abdominus:* This muscle arises by means of tendons from the crest of the pubis. The muscle inserts into the cartilages of the fifth, sixth, and seventh ribs, although this is quite variable.

　iii)　*Transversus Abdominus:* These muscles arise from the inner surface of ribs six through twelve. The fibers insert into the deepest layer of the abdominal aponeurosis.

　iv)　*External Obliques:* The external obliques take their origin from the exterior surfaces and lower borders of ribs 5 through 12. Some fibers terminate on the anterior half of the iliac crest and the rest terminate along the extent of the external layer of the abdominal aponeurosis.

　v)　*Internal Obliques:* The internal obliques arise from the lateral half of the inguinal ligament and from the anterior two-thirds of the iliac crest. They insert into the lower borders of the cartilages of the last three or four ribs.

(b)　**Secondary Muscles of Expiration:**
Secondary muscles of expiration are active under conditions of stress.

　i)　*Serratus Posterior Inferiorus:* These muscles originate at the aponeuroses of the spinous processes of thoracic vertebrae 11 and 12 and from lumbar vertebrae 1, 2, and 3. The fibers insert into the inferior borders of ribs 8 through 12, just lateral to angles.

ii) *Quadratus Lumborum:* These muscles originate at the aponeuroses of the iliac crest and at the ilio-lumbar ligament. They insert into the transverse processes of lumbar vertebrae 1 through 4 and into the medial half and lower border of the last rib.

iii) *Subcostals:* The subcostals have the same origins and insertions as the intercostals, but are distinguished from them because the subcostals generally are not confined to only one intercostal space.

iv) *Latissimus Dorsi:* These muscles originate from the spines of the lower t horacic vertebrae, the lumbar vertebrae, the sacrum, and from the posterior third of the iliac crest by means of a broad aponeurosis. They insert into the upper humerus by means of a stout tendon.

IV. **Measurement of Respiratory Function**

Speech-language pathologists are interested in respiratory function when evaluating causes of phonatory (voice) disorders. Respiratory efficiency is essential to vocal function. Phonatory function appears to be most efficient when airflow is steady, at midthoracic volumes.

A. **Spirometry**

One way respiratory function is measured is with a device called a spirometer. Spirometry provides a measure of how much air volume the respiratory system can move. There are other ways of gaining information about an individual's respiratory efficiency and vocal function without using instrumentation. They include measuring an individual's maximum phonation time, calculating the "s/z" ratio, and determining the resting respiratory rate.

B.   **Volumes**

1.   ***Vital Capacity:*** The total volume of air measured in cubic centimeters that can be exhaled after a maximum inspiration.

2.   ***Tidal Volume:*** The volume of air used in quiet breathing (Normal ~ 500 cc).

3.   ***Inspiratory Reserve (Complementary):*** The volume that can be inhaled beyond the tidal inspiration (Normal ~1600 cc).

4.   ***Expiratory Reserve (Supplementary):*** The volume that can be exhaled beyond tidal expiration (Normal ~1600 cc).

5.   ***Residual:*** The volume of air remaining in the lungs at maximum expiration. Air remains there because of the tendency of the ribs to pull away and hold the lungs open (Normal ~500 cc).

V.   **Diseases of the Respiratory System**

A.   **Asthma**

Asthma is a chronic condition of transient reversible attacks of respiratory distress. These attacks are characterized by spasm of the bronchial muscles, swelling of bronchial epithelium, and plugging of airways by mucous secretions. Various environmental and psychologic stimuli may trigger the attacks. Environmental stimuli include airborne allergens, viruses, medications, and cold air. Psychologic factors are associated with situational stressors.

B.   **Chronic Obstructive Pulmonary Disease (COPD)**

COPD is a collective term for a group of diseases involving obstruction of airflow or inhibition of the diffusion of gases through the alveoli. They include asthma, emphysema, chronic bronchitis, and others.

1.   ***Emphysema:*** Emphysema is a result of long-term distention of the alveoli with subsequent loss of tissue elasticity and poor osmotic gas transfer. As the condition progresses the number of alveoli decreases. Patients will exhibit a blushed complexion and rapid respiratory rate. The condition is irreversible and progressive resulting in death from right cardiac failure or massive infection.

2.   ***Chronic Bronchitis:*** Long-term inflammation of the bronchial tree is known as chronic bronchitis. This condition is marked by increased mucus production, tissue swelling, and subsequent scarring of the bronchial lining. This results in impeded airflow to

alveoli, although alveolar gas exchange is normal. Patients with chronic bronchitis often have a bluish complexion suggesting low blood oxygen content. They exhibit distinct respiratory sounds including rales (crackles) and ronchi (low wheezes). The condition is common in heavy cigarette smokers. Speech-language pathologists frequently encounter patients having chronic respiratory disease. Clinical intervention in such cases might include training in speech phrasing to make efficient use of limited respiratory volumes. Interdisciplinary coordination between attending physicians, nursing staff, inspiration, physical, occupational therapists, and other rehabilitation staff is also an important consideration.

UNIT 4

THE PHONATORY MECHANISM

I. **General Structure and Function**

A. **General Description and Location**

The larynx occupies the inferior part of the pharynx. This part of the pharynx is called the laryngopharynx. As the most inferior part of the pharynx, the larynx is part of the respiratory passages and forms a hollow tube to allow air to pass to and from the lungs. The larynx is specially developed to interrupt the flow of air. The larynx is a midline cervical structure with a multiply articulated, cartilaginous skeleton, an intrinsic muscular system, and a covering of several types of epithelium. It is located in the middle cervical area between the hyoid bone, superiorly, and the trachea, inferiorly. The larynx is anterior to the spine and esophagus.

B. **Evolution**

Phylogenetically lower animals also have larynges. These larynges are most primitive in amphibians (like the frog) and birds, but more developed in mammals like the dog. Although the dog's larynx is similar in function to the human larynx, the larynx in lower animals appears to be more for making sounds than for airway protection.

C. **Biological Function**

The primary function of the larynx is to protect the upper airway. It also can block escape of pulmonic air when we want to hold our breath, or when thoracic rigidity is important. For example, when we want to lift something heavy we inflate our chests, adduct our vocal folds, and lift. Thoracic rigidity is also required for defecation and during childbirth. In addition to those functions, the valve of the larynx helps to clear the airway by permitting air pressure to build up and produce an explosive release through coughing.

D. **Speech Function**

- The larynx provides the phonatory source for speech as well as the ability to produce glottal consonants. The phonatory source is a quasiperiodic sound created at the glottis. Glottal consonants include the glottal fricatives, /h/ and /ɦ/, and the glottal plosive, /ʔ/.

- Briefly, the voice is produced by rapid opening and closing of the glottal aperture. This action excites the air in the vocal tract and creates a resonating effect that is unique to the individual speaker. It is created when air is forced through the loosely adducted vocal folds which are opening and closing cyclically as a result of maintained muscle tension and aerodynamics. This cyclic opening and closing is called phonation. The glottal fricatives and plosives are produced just as other fricatives and plosives, except that the vocal tract constriction is at the glottis rather than the oral cavity.

1. **The Glottis and Vocal Folds**

   The space between the vocal folds is called the glottis, although some scientists consider the glottis to include the vocal folds. The glottis opens when air must pass to and from the lower respiratory tract and closes when the airway entrance must be closed or during phonation.

   a. **Abduction**

   When the vocal folds are held apart, they are said to be abducted. Abduction is accomplished by muscular action.

   b. **Adduction**

   Closed vocal folds are said to be adducted. Adduction is also accomplished by muscular action. The vocal folds are adducted during phonation. However, there is a brief open phase during the glottal cycle. This open phase is created by air pressure from the lower respiratory tract and is not considered abduction because it is not caused by muscular action.

2. **Physiology of Normal Phonation**

   a. **The Glottal cycle**

   The glottis opens and closes in successive phases during phonation. One opening and closing is referred to as the glottis cycle. After one cycle the process repeats itself until the speaker either decides to stop phonating or runs out of air (or both). Vocal physiologists have analyzed the glottal cycle to more fully understand phonation. On the most basic level, there are two phases to the cycle: a closed phase and an open phase. As you might imagine, the folds are held together during the closed phase and are driven apart during the open phase by subglottic air pressure.

   (1) **Closed Phase**

   During the closed phase the vocal folds are held in a loosely adducted posture. This posture will be maintained as long as the speaker intends to produce a voice, although it may change according to pitch and loudness requirements. Air pressure produced by relaxation of the muscles of inspiration, or sometimes contraction of the muscles of expiration, builds up inferior to the vocal folds and forces them open.

(2) **Open Phase**

The open phase can be broken down further into two parts: an opening phase, during which the folds are moving away from the midline under pressure from pulmonic air, and a closing phase.

(a) *Opening Phase:* As soon as there is the slightest opening between the folds, they are said to be in the open phase. It is important to stress that opening of the glottis during phonation is not a muscular action, but a function of aerodynamics.

(b) *Closing Phase:* During the closing phase, the vocal folds are moving back toward the midline. In this phase the vocal folds are under the influence of two forces: myoelasticity and the Bernoulli effect.

(3) **Forces**

(a) *Myoelastic:* Myoelasticity is the natural tendency of the muscles and tissues of the adducted vocal folds to resist deformation. The degree to which a muscle is contracted is referred to as its tonic status. As long as the tonic status of the muscles underlying the vocal folds is maintained; that is, the muscles are held loosely contracted, they will naturally tend to spring back to their original loosely adducted position once the air pressure has been relieved. This pressure starts to drop the instant the glottis opens.

(b) *Aerodynamic:* The Bernoulli effect (named for Swiss physicist, Daniel Bernouilli, 1738) is an aerodynamic principle which dictates a drop in the internal pressure of a fluid medium, such as air, as its velocity increases. It is the same principle that causes lift of an aircraft wing. Through the Bernoulli effect, the vocal folds are sucked back toward the midline once air begins to move between them. This action is aided by the natural tonus of the activated muscles of glottal adduction. The principle of phonatory glottal closing is called the Myoelastic-Aerodynamic Principle of Phonation. As soon as the vocal folds return to their loosely adducted position, air pressure begins to build. The entire glottal cycle then begins anew. Glottal cycles repeat many times per second until the speaker stops phonating. During the glottal cycle, little puffs of air are emitted up into the vocal tract by the rapid opening and closing of the glottis. These puffs excite the air in the tract, causing a nearly periodic complex tone. This tone is called either the glottal source, phonatory source, or the voice.

b. **Glottal Frequency**

(1) **Average Glottal Frequency**

The more openings and closings of the glottis during a given time (1 second), the higher we perceive the pitch of the speaker. Glottal (vocal) pitch is related to the frequency of the glottal cycle, or glottal frequency. Frequency is the number of times the glottal cycle repeats itself every second. It is measured in terms of cycles per second or hertz (Hz). The word hertz comes from the name of a famous physicist, Heinrich Hertz (1857–1894). It is important to stress that the perception of pitch is a psychological phenomenon related to the physical parameter of frequency.

(a) *Males:* The average fundamental frequency of a male voice is about 130 Hz.

(b) *Females:* The average fundamental frequency for a female voice is 250 Hz.

(2) **Mechanism for Changing Glottal Frequency**

A speaker can change glottal frequency by altering the length and tension of the vocal folds. When the vocal folds are stretched, their mass per unit of length is reduced and they move faster. Tension of the vocal folds is increased by the intrinsic laryngeal muscles: the cricothyroid and the thyroarytenoid muscles. The thyroarytenoid muscles are part of the mass of the vocal folds.

c. **Glottal Cycle Amplitude**

Loudness of the voice is associated with changes in the amplitude of the glottal cycle. Amplitude can refer to how far the folds are blown away from the midline or it can refer to the amount of particle displacement in the vocal tract air. The second interpretation is more pertinent. Until the middle of the previous century, it was thought that the farther apart the vocal folds are blown (the greater the amplitude of displacement and greater the area of the glottal aperture), the louder the voice (Zemlin, 1998). Recent research has found, however, that this is only the case in some speakers. For others, there is no difference in the distance of maximum vocal fold displacement. Rather, the mechanism for changing glottal cycle amplitude depends upon the coordinated action of the muscles of respiration and the muscles of glottal adduction. Respiratory forces increase subglottic pressure and glottal adductors increase vocal fold resistance. It is important to stress that loudness, like pitch, is a psychological phenomenon. Amplitude is the physical parameter.

II. The Framework of the Larynx

A. The Hyoid Bone

The hyoid bone is considered a bone of the skull; and, as such, it is part of the axial skeleton. It is situated just below the mandible.

1. **Structure**

The hyoid bone is shaped like a "U" or a horseshoe. It is open posteriorly and curved in the front. The hyoid bone has a body and two sets of projections called horns.

a. **Corpus:** This is the body of the hyoid. In Latin, corpus means body.

b. **Greater Cornua:** Cornu means horn. In this case, the horns are processes or projections of bone away from the body. The hyoid bone has two sets of horns. One pair is larger than the other and is called the greater cornua. The greater cornua come from the third branchial arch and project posteriorly from the corpus.

c. **Lesser Cornua:** The other smaller pair is called the lesser cornua. These project superiorly from the corpus and develop from the hyoid arch.

2. **Function of the Hyoid Bone**

   a. **Attachments**

   The hyoid bone serves as an attachment for many of the muscles of the head and neck, including the extrinsic muscles of the larynx. The extrinsic muscles of the larynx are those muscles that are attached to the larynx at one end and to something external to the larynx on the other end. Some of the muscles attached to the hyoid bone at one end are attached to the sternum and clavicles on the other end. The middle constrictor of the pharynx also attaches to the hyoid bone, as do the stylohyoid and mylohyoid muscles.

   b. **Relationship to Tongue and to Larynx**

   The hyoid bone provides inferior support to the tongue and superior support to the larynx. As the tongue and the larynx are freely movable, this relationship allows the muscles between them to function in various ways. For example, they can pull the larynx up, toward the tongue, or they can pull the tongue down, toward the larynx.

B. **Cartilages of the Larynx**

There are 11 cartilages in the larynx that can be divided into two groups: paired and unpaired. The unpaired laryngeal cartilages are single structures, located on the midline of the larynx. The paired laryngeal cartilages come in pairs and are located on either side of midline.

1. **Unpaired Cartilages of the Larynx**

   a. **Thyroid Cartilage**
   - The thyroid cartilage is suspended from the hyoid bone superiorly by ligaments and membranes. It articulates with the cricoid cartilage inferiorly. It surrounds the cricoid cartilage on three sides, anteriorly and laterally. Internally, the thyroid cartilage is the anterior attachment for the vocal ligaments. These vocal ligaments form the connective tissue infrastructure of the vocal folds. The vocal folds are attached to the interior aspects of the thyroid laminae from their anterior extent and all along their lateral margins.

- The thyroid cartilage is the largest laryngeal cartilage. It is the most readily palpated cartilage in your neck. Palpate means to touch and feel with your fingers.

(1)   **Structure**

  (a)   *Laminae:* The thyroid cartilage has two flat areas called laminae that are fused at the anterior midline to form the laryngeal prominence. This prominence is commonly called the Adam's apple, but the proper term is laryngeal prominence. The angle of fusion of these laminae is of significance. In males the angle is about 90 degrees. In females it may be up to 120 degrees. This angle may be significant in determining glottal frequency, as it brings the anterior attachment of the vocal ligament nearer the posterior as it increases. An anatomically shorter vocal ligament has less mass and may vibrate faster. There is a notch in the superior margin of the thyroid laminae with its deepest part at the point of their fusion. This is called the thyroid notch.

  (b)   *Cornua:* The thyroid cartilage has horns like the hyoid bone. These horns are called the horns inferior and superior and extend in those directions at the posterior margin of the laminae. The superior horns are attachments for ligaments that connect to the greater horns of the hyoid bone, superiorly. The inferior horns articulate with the cricoid cartilage with an amphiarthrodial joint at two articular facets on either side of the cricoid arch.

b.   **Cricoid Cartilage**

(1)   **Attachments**

The cricoid cartilage is the lowest cartilage of the larynx. It articulates with the thyroid cartilage laterally, with the arytenoid cartilages superiorly, and with the first tracheal ring inferiorly. The cricoid cartilage articulates with the thyroid cartilage at the inferior thyroid cornua laterally. The thyroid extends superiorly to the cricoid and the two are connected by a cricothyroid membrane. The cricoid cartilage is attached inferiorly to the first tracheal ring by means of a cricotracheal membrane.

(2) **Structure**

It is conventional to compare the shape of the cricoid cartilage to a signet ring. The cricoid cartilage is cylindrical, with its greatest height at its posterior aspect, and narrowing to a much shorter anterior part.

(a) *Lamina:* The lamina is the part of the ring on which your high school's name might be engraved. The cricoid cartilage has only one lamina, and it closes up the cricoid ring posteriorly. Some important attachments and articulations are with the lamina on its superior and posterior surfaces. The lamina is relatively flat posteriorly and, on its top margins, slopes gradually down in the anterior direction.

(b) *Arch:* Continuing the signet ring comparison, the cricoid arch would be the part that goes around under one's finger. Its superior surface slopes inferiorly from the lamina and becomes thinnest anteriorly. The paired arytenoid cartilages glide along this slope, accounting for the downward movement of the vocal folds upon adduction.

(c) *Articular Surfaces:* The articular surface of the cricoid lamina is located on its top and extends down onto the arch a bit. This is the smooth surface at which the arytenoid cartilages move. The joint between the cricoid lamina and the paired arytenoid cartilages is a very flexible amphiarthrodial joint by virtue of which the vocal folds can assume a variety of postures. On either side of the cricoid cartilage, just anterior to the lamina, is an articular surface for the thyroid cartilage. The rounded ends of the inferior thyroid cornua articulate at this point.

c.   **Epiglottis**

(1)   **Structure and Location**

The epiglottis is a flat, leaf-shaped, elastic carti-lage located at the base of the tongue. It projects posteriorly and superiorly away from the root of the tongue to which it is connected by loose epithelial tissue called the glossoepiglottic fold.

(2)   **Attachments of the Epiglottis**

The epiglottis is attached anteriorly to the hyoid bone corpus by means of a hyoepiglottic ligament. It is also attached to the thyroid cartilage by the thyroepiglottic ligament, just below the thyroid notch. The posterior and superior margin of the epiglottis is free.

(3)   **Glossoepiglottic Folds**

Stratified epithelium covers the entire inlet, including the epiglottis. There are mucous glands in this area, particularly on the posterior surface of the epiglottis. This epithelial tissue is elevated in three places forming the median and the lateral glossoepiglottic folds.

(a)   *Epiglottic Valleculae:* The bilateral spaces formed between the median and lateral glossoepiglottic folds are called the epiglottic valleculae. The epiglottic valleculae are important in the study of swal-lowing. If the extrinsic laryngeal muscles fail to function properly during swal-lowing, material may collect or pool in the valleculae. This is not uncommon following a cerebral vascular accident (CVA). If the pooled material remains in the valleculae after the swallow or the valleculae becomes too full before the swallow, material may enter the airway causing coughing or choking in attempts to expel it, or aspiration if the material enters the lower airway.

(b)   *Laryngeal Inlet:* The entrance to the larynx is called the laryngeal inlet, the additus, or the vestibule. This is where the digestive tract and airway separate.

(4)   **Epiglottitis**

If disease causes inflammation of the inlet mucosa around the epiglottis, the condition is called epiglottitis, and may become a medical emergency. Epiglottitis is a life-threatening condition due to the swollen tissues limiting the passage of air through the vocal tract.

2.   **Paired Cartilages of the Larynx**

a.   **Arytenoid Cartilages**

(1)   **Structure**

The arytenoid cartilages are roughly shaped like pyramids. These pyramids sit atop the cricoid cartilage, at the lamina, and their bases extend down along the upper edges of the arch. At the bottom (bases) of the arytenoid cartilages are the arytenoid processes.

(a)   *Vocal Processes:* The vocal processes of each arytenoid cartilage project anteriorly toward the inside of the thyroid laminae. They serve as the posterior attachments of the vocal ligaments. The joint between the arytenoids and cricoid cartilage is freely movable. The vocal ligaments can assume various postures by virtue of the fact that their posterior ends move about with the arytenoid cartilages.

(b)   *Muscular Processes:* The muscular processes of each arytenoid cartilage project laterally. They serve as the points of attachment of several intrinsicmuscles. Intrinsicmuscles have both attachments within the structure of the larynx.

(2)   **Function**

The articulation of the cricoid cartilage and the arytenoid cartilage is called the cricoarytenoid joint. The cricoarytenoid joint is freely movable and synovial. This means the arytenoid cartilages can move in several directions and, when they do, take the posterior part of the vocal ligaments with them.

Because the vocal ligament is the medial part of the vocal fold, the result is great variability in postural options for the vocal folds. Such options contribute to the ability of a speaker or singer to vary the voice. Note that, because the anterior ends of the vocal ligaments are attached to the inside of the single, unpaired thyroid cartilage, there will not be movement at the anterior end.

(a)   *Abduction/Adduction:* The gross function of the true vocal folds is opening and closing of the airway. To accomplish this, the arytenoid cartilages bring the posterior ends of the folds to and from the midline through contractions of the appropriate muscles. The manner and degree to which they do this is of interest to students of the voice.

   i)   **Rotation:** When the bases of the arytenoid cartilages rotate they cause the vocal processes to move to and from the midline.

   ii)   **Gliding or Sliding:** The arytenoid cartilages can slide laterally across the superior surface of the cricoid lamina, also moving the vocal processes to and from the midline.

   iii)   **Tilting:** The cartilages can tilt at their tops (apices), bringing the tips of the pyramids together or apart.

(b)   *Cartilaginous Glottis:* As the vocal ligament is attached posteriorly to the vocal processes of each arytenoid cartilage, the vocal processes form part of the space between the vocal folds. This part of the glottis is referred to as the cartilaginous glottis (Remember, the entire vocal folds, cartilage, muscle, and ligaments are covered by mucous membrane). We do not expect much movement from the cartilaginous portion of the glottis during phonation. It is relatively stiff, especially when the folds are adducted. The cartilaginous portion of the glottis occupies about one-third of its length, starting at its posterior end. Forceful adduction of the cartilaginous glottis can result in a painful contact ulcer.

(c) *Membranous Glottis:* The rest of the glottis is called the membranous glottis and takes up two-thirds of glottal length. Normal glottal opening and closing during phonation takes place in the anterior two-thirds of the glottis.

b. **Minor Paired Cartilages of the Larynx**

There are several minor cartilages of the larynx. These are vestigial structures and probably serve to give structure to the connective tissue of the larynx. They are all paired and are located between the arytenoid apices and the hyoid bone.

(1) **Corniculate Cartilages**

These cartilages are located within the aryepiglottic folds, superior and posterior to the apices of each arytenoid cartilage. Because the arytenoid apexes tilt posteriorly anyway, the corniculate cartilages look like continuations of the tips of the arytenoid cartilages.

(2) **Cuneiform Cartilages**

A little farther up from where the corniculate cartilages are located in the aryepiglottic folds are two more minor cartilages: the cuneiform cartilages. Not everyone has cuneiform cartilages.

(3) **Triticeal Cartilages**

Triticeal cartilages are not much more than cartilaginous lumps in the lateral thyrohyoid ligaments located between the superior horns of the thyroid cartilage and the greater horns of the hyoid bone.

C. **Ligaments of the Larynx**

1. **Extrinsic Ligaments**

Extrinsic ligaments attach to the larynx at one end and to some structure outside the larynx at the other end. As there are only two ends of the larynx, there are only two extrinsic ligaments.

a.   **Thyrohyoid Ligament**

The thyrohyoid membrane and ligaments attach the thyroid cartilage and the rest of the larynx (as the thyroid cartilage is connected to the rest of the larynx) to the hyoid bone. It is important to remember that the hyoid bone is not a part of the larynx. Thus, the thyrohyoid ligament is extrinsic because it attaches at one end to the hyoid bone. It follows the horizontal U-shaped outline of the hyoid bone and the thyroid cartilage and is open posteriorly. At its midline front and at its two rear ends, laterally, the thyrohyoid membrane is thicker than in other portions. These three points are referred to as thyrohyoid ligaments. The two posterolateral sections are referred to as the lateral thyrohyoid ligaments and the anteromedial section is called the median thyrohyoid ligament. The lateral and posterior portions connect the superior horns of the thyroid cartilage with the posterior ends of the greater horns of the hyoid bone. Recall that the triticeal cartilages are contained within the lateral thyrohyoid ligaments. Between the thickened portions, the connective tissue becomes thin and is called the thyrohyoid membrane. There is a distinctive hole (aperture) in the thyrohyoid membrane through which the superior laryngeal nerve, artery, and vein pass.

b.   **Cricotracheal Ligament**

The larynx is attached to the trachea at its inferior end, so the ligament that attaches the cricoid cartilage to the first tracheal ring is called the cricotracheal ligament. The flexibility of the cricotracheal ligament and of the respiratory cartilages allows movement of these structures during breathing and as the individual assumes various postures.

2.   **Intrinsic Ligaments**

Intrinsic membranes and ligaments attach to the larynx at both ends. There are several of these, but the most significant one is the conus elasticus. To a certain extent, students may consider that the membranes extending within the larynx from inferior to superior are all parts of one expanse of dense connective tissue with a few gaps in the ventricular region.

a.   **Conus Elasticus (Cricovocal Membrane)**

The term conus elasticus refers to a structure of dense connective tissue which shapes the subglottic area. This membrane forms a cone and the empty space in the middle of it is called the subglottic space. The conus elasticus is a membrane composed of two thicker parts (ligaments): one on the superior surface and one on its anterior surface. The superior free border is the thick vocal ligament. The vocal ligament is the skeleton (medial portion) of the vocal folds. The anterior, medial part of the conus elasticus is also thick and is called the cricothyroid ligament. It attaches superiorly to the thyroid cartilage where the laminae fuse (Adam's apple) and inferiorly to the upper border of the cricoid arch. The whole structure that forms into these thicker ligaments follows along the cricoid arch and is called the conus elasticus. The conus elasticus forms an anatomic irregular cone open at the top and bottom through which pulmonary air passes during speech. It is the shape of this cone that enables the Bernoulli effect to suck the vocal folds closed during phonation.

b. **Vocal Ligament**

The upper free border of the conus elasticus forms the vocal ligaments. These ligaments come together in the front at their attachments to the inner lamina of the thyroid cartilage. Posteriorly, they attach to the bases of the two arytenoid cartilages. Remember, they extend inferiorly into the conus elasticus. The vocal ligaments form the inner connective tissue framework of the vocal folds. In front, its two ends are attached to the inner aspect of the thyroid cartilage, near the point at which the laminae fuse. There, they have a single point of attachment. The posterior attachments of the vocal ligaments are the vocal processes of the two arytenoid cartilages. Because the articulation between the cricoid and arytenoid cartilages is diarthroidal, the vocal folds can move freely with the arytenoid's at their posterior ends. Anteriorly, they are fixed to the inner thyroid angle.

c. **Cricothyroid Ligament**

The anterior and medial part of the conus elasticus is also thick and is called the cricothyroid ligament. It attaches superiorly to the thyroid cartilage where the laminae fuse (Adam's apple) and inferiorly to the upper border of the cricoid arch. Its importance lies in the fact that it is anatomically part of the vocal ligament.

d. **Vestibular Ligament**

The vestibular ligament is attached to the thyroid cartilage anteriorly, and to the arytenoid apices posteriorly. It may be considered the superior version of the vocal ligament. It forms the connective tissue infrastructure of two weaker ventricular (vestibular) folds, separating the vestibule above, from the ventricle below.

III.   **Articulations of the Larynx**

A.   **Cricothyroid Articulation**

1.   **Rotation About the Horizontal Axis**
- The cricothyroid muscles act on both the cricoid and the thyroid cartilages, moving each in relationship to the other. There are two parts to the cricothyroid muscle: the pars recta (anterior) and pars oblique (lateral). When the pars recta contracts it rotates the thyroid and/or cricoid cartilages about a transverse axis through the cricothyroid joint. When the pars oblique contracts it pulls the thyroid cartilage forward in relationship to the cricoid.
- As the vocal ligament is firmly attached to the inside of the thyroid cartilage at one end and to the arytenoid cartilages at the other end, and the arytenoid cartilages are attached to the cricoid cartilages, it should be apparent that both actions increase vocal ligament tension. For this reason, and because it lies outside the laryngeal cavity, the cricothyroid muscle is sometimes called the external tensor. Tensing the cricothyroid muscles increase the pitch of the voice.

2.   **Gliding**

When, the pars oblique contracts, it pulls the thyroid cartilage forward in relation to the cricoid, further stretching or tensing the vocal ligament.

B.   **Cricoarytenoid Articulation**

1.   **Rotation**

The posterior cricoarytenoid muscles originate on either side of the cricoid lamina, posterior and inferior to the cricoarytenoid joints. Their fibers insert into the muscular process of each arytenoid cartilage. When the posterior cricoarytenoid muscles contract, they draw the muscular processes of the arytenoid cartilages posteriorly and inferiorly, rotating the arytenoid cartilages so that their vocal processes move away from the midline and slightly upward. This action abducts the vocal folds, opening the glottis for respiration or for articulation of voiceless speech sounds. The posterior cricoarytenoid muscles are the only vocal fold abductors.

2. **Gliding or Sliding (Anterior/Posterior and Lateral/Medial)**

- The lateral cricoarytenoid muscles act in opposition to the posterior cricoarytenoid muscles. They originate on the lateral aspects of the cricoid arch, anterior and inferior to the artyenoid cartilages, and insert on the muscular processes of each arytenoid cartilage. When the fibers of the lateral cricoarytenoid muscles contract, they draw the muscular processes of the arytenoid cartilages anteriorly and downward, rotating the arytenoid cartilages on their vertical axes so that the vocal processes move medially. This closes the glottal aperture.

- The transverse arytenoid muscle is the only unpaired intrinsic laryngeal muscle. Fibers are attached to each arytenoid cartilage on their posterior and lateral aspects from base to apex. Contraction of these fibers draws the two arytenoid cartilages together, sliding them medially across the top of the cricoid lamina and tightening glottal closure.

3. **Tilting**

The paired oblique arytenoid muscle fibers form a thin muscle that stretches from the base of one arytenoid cartilage to the apex of the other. They cross each other and are superficial to the transverse arytenoid muscles. Contraction of oblique arytenoid fibers tilts the apices of the arytenoid cartilages together.

IV. **Cavities of the Larynx (Laryngopharynx)**

A. **Vestibular (Superior) Division**

This is the entrance of the larynx. It is protected by the aryepiglottic folds and the epiglottis itself. The vestibule extends from inlet to the ventricular folds. The ventricular folds are called either ventricular or vestibular, depending on whether you think of them as being in the superior division or in the middle division of the laryngeal cavity. The most prominent feature of the vestibular division is the eminence in the aryepiglottic fold created by the epiglottis.

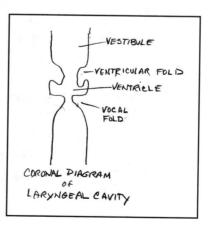

1. *Location and Extent:* Vestibular division extends from the inlet to the ventricular folds.

2. *Epiglottis:* Protects the inlet.

3. *Aryepiglottic Folds:* Mucosa that covers the epiglottis and extends inferiorly to the arytenoid cartilages.

B.   Ventricular (Middle Division)

1. **Location and Extent:** From Ventricular (Vestibular) Folds to Vocal Folds.

2. **Ventricular Folds**

    It is possible to adduct and excite the air in the pharynx with pulses generated by the ventricular folds. This is not a normal phonation and sounds very rough. Some people phonate in this pathologic way. The condition is called dysphonia plica ventricularis.

    a. **Composition**

        Soft and flaccid, the ventricular folds are composed of thin muscle covered with mucous membrane.

    b. **Attachments**

        The ventricular folds attach to the anterolateral surface of arytenoid cartilages posteriorly near the triangular fovea of each arytenoid cartilage. Anteriorly, they are more prominent. They attach to the inner surface of the thyroid cartilage about where the epiglottis attaches. The ventricular folds are sometimes called the false vocal folds, and the space between the ventricular folds is sometimes called the false glottis because of their role in producing an abnormal voice source.

3. **Vocal Folds**

    The vocal folds produce the normal voice. They are located inferior to ventricular folds. It is customary among some speech-language pathologists to refer to these folds as the true vocal folds.

    a. **Composition**

        Each vocal fold is a bundle of muscle tissue and a vocal ligament covered by epithelial tissue. There are four layers of epithelium, which vary in consistency from a stiff, squamous, capsular form to an almost jellylike loose epithelium. The vocal ligament is the upper free border of the conus elasticus or cricovocal membrane.

(1)   **Thyroarytenoid Muscles**

- Thyroarytenoid muscles attach to the inner surface of the thyroid cartilage anteriorly and laterally, and to the bases of each arytenoid cartilage posteriorly. When they contract, they can stiffen the vocal folds or draw the arytenoid cartilages anteriorly and their lateral (thyromuscularis) fibers can adduct the vocal folds by acting on the muscular processes of the arytenoid cartilages.

- The muscular portion of the vocal folds includes the thyroarytenoid muscles and the vocalis muscles. The vocalis muscles are situated immediately lateral to the vocal ligaments.

(2)   **Vocalis Muscles**

Myographic studies suggest there are distinct medial muscle bundles called the vocalis muscles, sometimes called the internal thyroarytenoid muscles. This is important physiologically, as thyroarytenoid muscles may be contracted separately from the vocalis muscles, leaving the vocalis muscle masses loose and free to vibrate on their own. This produces a very high pitch voice, as the vocalis mass is much less than that of the whole focal fold. This high-frequency voice is known as falsetto.

(3)   **Vocal Ligaments**

The vocal ligaments form the skeletal structure for the inner (medial) portions of the vocal folds.

(4)   **Soft Tissue Layers**

The superficial layer is stratified squamous epithelium with its basement membrane. Deep to this are three layers of lamina propria. The deepest part of a vocal fold is the vocal ligament.

b.   **Attachments and Positioning of the Vocal Folds**

Attachments of the vocal folds are the same as those for the thyroarytenoid muscles. They attach to the thyroid cartilage anteriorly and laterally and to the bases of the arytenoids posteriorly.

4. **Glottis**

The glottis is the space between the vocal folds. In some anatomy texts you will read that the glottis includes the vocal folds and the space, with the name rima glottis applied specifically to the space. Part of this space is occupied by the vocal processes of the arytenoid cartilages and the rest by the vocal ligament. Specialists in vocal function, including some speech-language pathologists, have studied glottal anatomy and physiology to the extent that they have divided the glottis into parts.

a. **Intermembranous**

- The intermembranous portion of the glottis is supported by the vocal ligament. This portion occupies the anterior two-thirds of the glottal opening. With its anterior and posterior ends fixed in place by their attachments to cartilages, the part between the cartilages is relatively free to vibrate during phonation, opening and closing with each glottal cycle.

- The midpoint of the intermembranous glottis has the least mechanical support. As you might imagine, the midpoint is the part that tends to move farthest away from the sagittal plane during optimal phonation. This point is called the point of maximum excursion by vocal physiologists. Interestingly, the point of maximum excursion moves anteriorly as glottal frequency is raised, and posteriorly when frequency is lowered. Because the most mechanically efficient location for the point of maximum excursion is at the midpoint of the intermembranous glottis, habitually speaking with this point too far away from the midpoint will cause strain on the vocal mechanism.

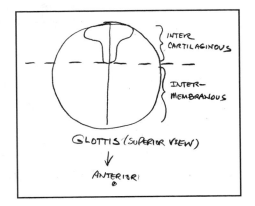

b. **Intercartilaginous**

The intercartilaginous portion of the glottis is supported by the vocal processes of the arytenoid cartilages. This portion occupies the posterior one-third of the glottal opening. It is relatively stiff and does not vibrate like the intermembranous sides of the glottis.

C. Infraglottic (Subglottic) Division

Infraglottic (subglottic) division is the space immediately inferior to the vocal folds. This is the area where pulmonic air pressure is increased to drive the phonatory source. Increases in subglottic air pressure attend increases in phonatory loudness. The conus elasticus covers the epithelium of the subglottic division, and its shape contributes to the generation of the Bernoulli effect during the glottal cycle.

V. Muscles of the Larynx: Intrinsic and Extrinsic

A. Intrinsic Muscles of the Larynx

While extrinsic muscles have an attachment outside the larynx, intrinsic muscles have origins and insertions located within the laryngeal organ. Intrinsic muscles of the larynx have three basic functions: (1) to control the length and tension of the vocal ligament; (2) to control the degree of glottal opening; and (3) to modify the opening of the laryngeal inlet. All but one of the intrinsic laryngeal muscles comes in pairs, one right and one left. Only the transverse arytenoid muscle is a singleton.

1. Muscles That Control Tension/Length of the Vocal Ligament

Changes in tension of the vocal ligaments, and hence the vocal folds, can strengthen glottal closure. For speech purposes, increasing vocal fold tension is accompanied by an increase in glottal frequency (i.e., an increase in perceived pitch).

a. Cricothyroid

As the name indicates, the cricothyroid muscles originate on either side of the cricoid arch and insert on each side of the thyroid laminae. When the cricothyroid muscles are shortened, their points of attachment are brought together. The cricothyroid muscle fibers insert on the thyroid cartilage in two sections. One section, called the pars recta, has a nearly vertical course and inserts on the lower part of the posterior thyroid lamina. The other fiber group has an oblique course and inserts on the inferior thyroid cornua. This group is called the pars oblique. In addition to the pars recta and pars oblique, a third group, the pars interna has been identified (Charpied, 2007).

b. Thyroarytenoid

Thyroarytenoid muscle fibers originate at several sites: (1) anteriorly and laterally, along the inner aspect of the thyroid laminae from their fusion and along the sides laminae; and (2) medially from the cricovocal membrane. Insertion is on the anterolateral aspect of the arytenoid cartilage bases.

c.   **Vocalis**

The thyroarytenoid muscles have a distinct medial bundle of fibers at their medial aspects where they attach to the cricovocal membrane. These medial fibers form muscle masses that are sometimes called the vocalis muscles or the medial (internal) thyroarytenoid muscles. The vocalis muscles can be tensed or relaxed independent of the lateral thyroarytenoid muscles.

2.   **Muscles That Control Glottal Aperture**

Opening and closing the glottal aperture have both biological and speech functions. Both functions require either opening (vocal fold abduction) or closing (vocal fold adduction) of the glottis. For biological purposes, an open glottal aperture is required to admit air into the respiratory system. At least six millimeters is sufficient for quiet breathing without exertion. During heavy breathing, the vocal folds are widely abducted and pressed against the walls of the laryngopharyngeal cavity. On expiration, the glottal aperture closes slightly. This maintains air in the lungs a little longer, facilitating gas exchange. For speech, the vocal folds are adducted loosely during phonation. All American English phonemes, except the voiceless obstruent consonants, require the presence of vibrating focal folds.

a.   **Posterior Cricoarytenoid:** These muscles originate on either side of the cricoid lamina, posterior and inferior to the cricoarytenoid joints. Their fibers insert into the muscular process of each arytenoid cartilage. When the posterior cricoarytenoid muscles contract, they draw the muscular processes of the arytenoid cartilages posteriorly and inferiorly. This movement rotates the arytenoid cartilages so that their vocal processes move away from the midline and slightly upward. This action abducts the vocal folds, opening the glottis for respiration or for articulation of voiceless speech sounds. The posterior cricoarytenoid muscles are the only vocal fold abductors.

b.   **Lateral Cricoarytenoid:** The lateral arytenoid muscles act in opposition to the posterior cricoarytenoid muscles. They originate on the lateral aspects of the cricoid arch, anterior and inferior to the artyenoid cartilages, and insert on the muscular processes of each arytenoid cartilage. When the fibers of the lateral cricoarytenoid muscles contract, they draw the arytenoids muscular processes anteriorly and downward. This movement rotates the arytenoid cartilages on their vertical axes causing the vocal processes to move medially and closing the glottal aperture.

c. **Transverse Arytenoid:** The transverse arytenoid muscle is the only unpaired intrinsic laryngeal muscle. Fibers are attached to each arytenoid cartilage on their posterior and lateral aspects, from base to apex. Contraction of these fibers draws the two arytenoid cartilages together, sliding them medially across the top of the cricoid lamina and tightening glottal closure.

d. **Oblique Arytenoid:** The paired oblique arytenoid muscle fibers form a thin muscle that stretches from the base of one arytenoid cartilage to the apex of the other. They cross each other and are superficial to the transverse arytenoid muscles. Contraction of the oblique arytenoid fibers tilt the apices of the arytenoid cartilages together.

3. **Muscles That Modify Laryngeal Inlet**

a. **Aryepiglottic:** The aryepiglottic muscle is a thin muscle which is embedded within the aryepiglottic fold. It is a circular continuation of the oblique arytenoid muscles. The aryepiglottic muscle assists in drawing the fold together in a sphincteric action to close the laryngeal inlet.

b. **Thyroepiglottic:** The thyroepiglottic muscles are continuations of the thyroarytenoid muscles. They extend from the thyroid cartilage to the epiglottis and draw those two structures together.

c. **Ventricular:** Within the flaccid ventricular folds are thin ventricular muscles. These can stiffen the ventricular folds slightly.

B. **Extrinsic Muscles of the Larynx**

Extrinsic muscles of the larynx control the posture of the larynx in relationship to other structures of the head and neck. They play a role in swallowing and in pharyngeal resonance. Their role in resonance means that both intrinsic and extrinsic muscles have roles in the sound of the voice. The extrinsic muscles can be grouped according to their location in relationship to the larynx and the hyoid bone.

1.   **Suprahyoid Muscles:** These muscles are called suprahyoid because they are positioned superior to the hyoid bone. In that location they cannot be proper extrinsic muscles because one of their ends cannot possibly be attached to the larynx. However, they are grouped with extrinsic laryngeal muscles by convention because they play a role in the positioning of the larynx. When the hyoid bone is elevated, and the muscles that attach the thyroid cartilage to the hyoid bone are fixed, then the larynx will elevate with the hyoid bone. However, they are not attached to the larynx because the hyoid bone is not part of the larynx. The suprahyoid extrinsic laryngeal muscles are listed below.

   a.   **Digastric**

   This is the only extrinsic laryngeal muscle whose name does not indicate its location. The name digastric means "two bellies." This muscle consists of one anterior belly and one posterior belly. The two bellies are joined by an intermediate tendon, attached to the hyoid corpus by a band of connective tissue. The anterior belly originates at the inside of the mandible, near the symphysis. The posterior belly originates deep to the mastoid process of the temporal bone. When both bellies contract in unison, they elevate the hyoid bone.

   b.   **Stylohyoid**

   This muscle originates at the styloid process, a thin bony projection just deep and inferior to the external auditory meatus. It inserts on the hyoid bone, where the intermediate tendon of the digastric muscle is located. At this location the stylohyoid muscle divides into two sections on either side of the digastric tendon. When the stylohyoid muscle contracts it draws the hyoid bone toward the styloid process, that is, back and up.

   c.   **Mylohyoid**

   This pair of muscles originates at a line on the medial surface of the mandible called the mylohyoid line. It inserts on the hyoid corpus and a medial connective tissue raphe, which separates the two mylohyoid muscles medially. The mylohyoid muscles form the floor of the anterior oral cavity. During the act of swallowing, the mylohyoid muscles push the tongue upward to help propel the food bolus or liquid volume posteriorly. The mylohyoid can also help open the mouth against resistance.

d. **Geniohyoid**

The geniohyoid muscle originates at the medial surface of the mandible at about the same place as the anterior belly of the digastric muscle, that is, right in the center of the medial mandibular surface, behind the chin, or mental eminence. The geniohyoid muscle, however, is located deep to the mylohyoid muscle, whereas the anterior diagastric belly is superficial to the mylohyoid. The two geniohyoid muscles insert on the anterior part of the hyoid corpus.

e. **Hyoglossus**

The hyoglossus muscles are rather flat and quadrilateral in shape. Because both ends of these muscles are attached to movable structures, it is difficult to designate an origin or insertion. One end of a hyoglossus muscle is attached to the lateral part of the tongue near the blade, and the other end is attached to a greater cornu of the hyoid. When a hyoglossus muscle contracts, it pulls one side of the tongue toward the hyoid bone or the hyoid bone up toward the tongue.

2. **Infrahyoid**

Infrahyoid muscles are situated inferior to the hyoid bone. The thyrohyoid and the sternothryoid are actually attached to the larynx. The others attach to the hyoid bone at their superior ends and to another structure at the other end. When they contract they can depress the hyoid bone, thus lowering the larynx, or they can directly depress the larynx.

a. ***Sternohyoid:*** The sternohyoid originates from the posterior portion of the manubrium of the sternum and the medial portion of the clavicle. It passes superiorly to insert on the lower border of the body of the hyoid bone (hyoid corpus). When the sternohyoid muscle contracts it pulls the hyoid bone inferiorly, toward the sternum.

b. ***Omohyoid:*** This muscle has two bellies, which, like the digastric muscles, are connected by a central tendon. The two bellies are called the superior belly and the inferior belly. The superior belly passes downward from the body of the hyoid bone to its intermediate tendon. The inferior belly passes from the deep surface of the scapula to the intermediate tendon. When the omohyoid muscles contract, they draw the hyoid bone toward the scapula.

c.   ***Thyrohyoid:*** The thyrohyoid muscle is attached to the thyroid cartilage lamina at one end, and to the greater cornu of the hyoid bone at the other end. It can draw the hyoid bone inferiorly toward the larynx or, depending upon which structure is fixed in place, draw the larynx superiorly toward the hyoid bone.

d.   ***Sternothyroid:*** The sternothyroid muscles originate on the sternum at the manubrium, and insert on the thyroid cartilage laminae. They draw the thyroid cartilage and the larynx inferiorly toward the sternum.

3.   **Indirect Displacers of the Larynx**

Indirect laryngeal displacers are extrinsic laryngeal muscles that move the larynx by acting on the pharyngeal tube.

a.   ***Palatopharyngeus:*** The palatopharyngeus muscle forms the bulk of the posterior faucial arch. It is attached at one end to the connective tissue aponeurosis of the velum as well as to the posterior part of the palatine bone. At its other end, it inserts into the fibers of the middle pharyngeal constrictor muscle. When it contracts it can either pull the velum inferiorly or pull the lateral walls of the pharynx superiorly.

b.   ***Stylopharyngeus:*** Stylopharyngeus muscles originate on the styloid process of the temporal bone and insert into the lateral pharyngeal walls between the superior and middle pharyngeal constrictors. They pull the pharyngeal wall up and to the rear.

c.   ***Inferior Pharyngeal Constrictor:*** The inferior pharyngeal constrictor is a nearly tubular muscle which forms the inferior part of the muscular pharynx. It originates at a median raphe extending vertically along its posterior aspect. Anteriorly, its fibers are attached to the cricoid and thyroid cartilages. When the fibers contract the entire larynx is pulled posteriorly. Tension of the pharyngeal constrictor muscles can alter the resonating characteristics of the vocal tract.

UNIT 5

THE ARTICULATORY MECHANISM

I.   **General Structure and Function of the Vocal Tract**

A.   **Structure**

1.   **Oral Cavity**

The oral cavity is formed by the space between the mandible and the maxilla. It is a highly variable and flexible opening, serving three functions. Two of these functions are biological: nutrition (hydration) and respiration. The third function is to modify the resonance of the laryngeal tone and to add two other sound sources for the articulation of speech. The vocal tract has been referred to as a multiple band-pass acoustic filter because of the way it resonates sound for speech.

a.   *Tongue:* The most prominent structure of the oral cavity is the tongue. It is very flexible and functions in swallowing and the articulation of speech. The tongue is composed of muscle and mucosal epithelium supported by a ligamentous connective tissue skeleton.

b.   *Dental Arches:* Two dental arches are seated in the superior (maxillary) and inferior (mandibular) alveolar processes. Their primary function is the mastication of food. Only the upper arch is used in speech and the upper incisors are the only teeth used for articulation.

c.   *Hard Palate:* The hard palate is so called to distinguish it from the velum, or soft palate. It is composed of mucosal epithelium covering bones of the facial skeleton: the palatal processes of each maxilla and the horizontal processes of each palatine bone. The hard palate serves as a hard surface for bolus manipulation or for generating negative pressure in sucking, as well as for speech articulation.

d.   *Velum (Soft Palate):* The velum, also known as the soft palate, forms the roof of the posterior oral cavity. It is composed of the same mucosal epithelial tissue that covers the hard palate. Its infrastructure is muscular. The muscles of the velum are the tensor veli palatini, levator veli palatini, palatoglossus, palatopharyngeus, and uvularis. The velum is part of the velopharyngeal sphincter, a muscular valve that separates and couples the nasopharynx with the rest of the vocal tract. When the velum is elevated, the resonance of the vocal tract is said to be oral; when it is depressed the resonance is said to be nasal. Speech that has too much nasal resonance is said to be hypernasal, whereas speech with too little nasal resonance is said to be hyponasal. The velopharyngeal sphincter may also seal off the nasopharynx during sucking and swallowing. The dimensions of the skull in infancy allow the velopharyngeal sphincter to remain open during swallowing. Neonates can breathe while nursing without danger of aspiration.

2. **Nasal Cavity**

The nasal cavity is a pair of twin openings superior to the oral cavity. It is rigid and not nearly as capable of modification as the oral cavity. Its rigidity ensures a patent opening to the respiratory tract. Its speech function is the addition of nasal resonance. It also houses the end organs for the sense of smell.

a. *Nares:* The nares are the anterior openings of the nasal cavity. They are sometimes called nostrils.

b. *Choanae:* The choanae are the posterior openings of the nasal cavity that lead into the nasopharynx.

c. *Septum:* The nasal passages are separated by a wall of bone and cartilage called the nasal septum. The septum is formed of bone at its posterior end and by cartilage at its anterior end.

3. **Pharyngeal Cavity**

The pharyngeal cavity extends from first tracheal ring to the posterior opening of the nasal cavity.

a. *Laryngopharynx*: The laryngopharynx extends from the laryngeal inlet to the first tracheal ring. It lies behind and partially around the larynx, which is its principal structure.

b. *Oropharynx*: The oropharynx extends from the inferior extent of the nasopharynx to the inlet of the larynx. It lies posterior to the buccal cavity, inferior to the soft palate, and superior to the inlet of the larynx. The faucial arches are the theoretical boundary between the oral cavity and the oropharynx.

c. *Nasopharynx*: The nasopharynx is the part of the pharynx which extends from the choanae to a plane reaching from the posterior portion of the hard palate to the pharyngeal wall. That is, the inferior end of the nasopharynx could be marked by drawing a line from the hard palate posteriorly to the pharyngeal wall.

B.   **Function**

1.   **Plosive and Fricative Sources for Obstruent Consonants**

Articulation of obstruent consonants is accomplished by juxtaposition of two structures in the vocal tract. These structures do not have to be located in the oral cavity. For example, the glottal fricative is articulated in the laryngopharynx.

2.   **Analogy to Band-Pass Filter for Vowels and Semivowels**

Vowels and approximants are produced by changing the shape of the muscles of the articulatory mechanism, thus changing the shape of the vocal tract interior. These sounds are produced with a more open vocal tract posture. A speaker can "play" the vocal tract like a musical instrument, moving the tongue up and down or forward and backward, and rounding or spreading the lips, and thereby changing the way the tract resonates in response to the vibration of the vocal folds (the phonatory source).

3.   **General Function**

During respiration air is usually taken in through the nasal cavity. The oral cavity provides an alternative opening. Air enters the pharynx because the velum is lowered by relaxing the muscles of velar elevation. Airflow continues through the laryngopharynx and into the trachea via the abducted vocal folds. Nutrition and hydration is accomplished via the oral cavity under normal circumstances. Material is prepared in the oral cavity and transferred posteriorly into the pharynx by manipulation of the mandible and tongue. The velum may be elevated to maintain intraoral pressure and to prevent nasal reflux. After entering the pharynx, the material is directed into the esophagus by elevation and obturation of the laryngeal inlet.

II.   **The Skull in General**

A.   **Gross Structure**

1.   **Skull**

a.   *Cranium:* The cranium consists of all the bones of the skull with the exception of the mandible (lower jaw) and the hyoid bone. The bones of the cranium include the frontal, parietal, occipital, temporal (with ossicles), sphenoid, ethmoid, lacrimal, inferior nasal concha, palatine, vomer, maxilla, zygomatic, and nasal. The cranium has two subdivisions: facial skeleton and calvaria.

(1) *Facial Skeleton:* This is the lower, anterior part of the skull. Several bones form the facial skeleton in addition to the mandible. These include the frontal, sphenoid, maxilla, lacrimal, ethmoid, inferior nasal concha, nasal, palatine, vomer, and zygomatic bones. Some of the bones of the facial skeleton form the structure underlying what we think of as the face.

(2) *Calvaria:* These bones form the bowl that protects the brain. The bones of the calvaria are the frontal, parietal, sphenoid, temporal, and occipital bones.

b. *Mandible:* The mandible is the lower jaw. It articulates with the temporal bone at a synovial joint called the temporomandibular joint.

c. *Hyoid bone:* Although it is most commonly associated with the larynx, the hyoid is a skull bone. It does not articulate with any other bone. It is located below the mandible and attaches by muscle and connective tissue to the root of the tongue, the mandible, epiglottis, pharynx, and the temporal bone.

2. **Cavities of the Cranium**

a. *Cranial Cavity:* The cranial cavity which houses the brain is formed by all the bones of the skull with the exception of the mandible. The cranial bones include the frontal, parietal, occipital, temporal, sphenoid, ethmoid, lacrimal, inferior nasal concha, palatine, vomer, maxilla, zygomatic, and nasal bones.

b. *Orbits:* The oral cavity does not exist without the mandible to form its inferior aspect. This familiar cavity is inferior to the nasal cavity in the midline of the face. It is the entrance to the digestive tract, an alternative entrance to the airway, and the location of most of the speech articulators. Its skeleton is formed by the mandible, maxillae, and palatine bones.

c.   ***Nasal Cavity:*** The nasal cavity is in the middle of the facial skeleton. It is the main entrance to the airway, seat of the organ of smell, and serves as an alternative vent and resonating cavity for speech. It is formed by the nasal and ethmoid bones, sphenoid, maxillae, vomer, and palatine bones, and inferior nasal conchae.

B.   **Bone Type**

The bones of the skull are specialized to help perform their protective function. Most of them, particularly the ones of the calvaria, are laminated like plywood. The outer layer is called the outer lamina. The inner layer is the inner lamina. The two laminae are separated by a spongy layer called diploe. The skull is exposed to a variety of mechanical stresses. Intrinsic forces are generated by the skull itself. Extrinsic forces are generated by outside pressures.

C.   **Mechanical Stresses**

Most forces that act on the skull are generated from the outside (extrinsic forces), but one force is generated intrinsically by exertion of the muscles of mastication on the mandible against the maxilla. This intrinsic force is usually applied along the line formed by the second upper molar, the zygomatic bone, the lateral margin of the orbit, and into the anterior calvaria. This force can be the source of some chronic pain. Extrinsic forces can be applied through sudden deceleration from outside the calvaria. They can also be applied along the vertebral column into the basal area of the skull through the basal portion of the occipital bone.

III.   **Superior Aspect of the Cranium**

A.   **Calvaria**

1.   **Frontal Bone**

In the anterior area of the calvaria is the frontal bone. During infancy the frontal bone is divided by a (metropic) suture, but it calcifies to produce an unpaired bone. The frontal bone forms the forehead and part of the orbits. From above we can observe that it articulates with the paired parietal bones.

2.   **Temporal Bones**

The temporal bones form parts of the lateral and basal aspects of the cranium. Anteriorly, they serve as attachments for several pharyngeal muscles and ligaments and contain articular facets for the mandible. Laterally, the temporal bones contain the structures of the ears.

3. **Sphenoid Bone**

The single sphenoid bone is located in the lower, middle part of the cranial cavity, posterior to the nasal cavity. It forms the superior skeletal infrastructure of the nasopharynx. The pteryoid muscle and tensor veli palatini muscles originate on the sphenoid bone. Only two small parts of the sphenoid ("the greater wings") bone contribute to the calvaria.

4. **Parietal Bones**

The paired parietal bones form the lateral and middle area of the upper skull. From the top we can see that the parietal bones articulate with the frontal bone. They do this at the coronal suture. They also articulate with the occipital bone in the rear at the lambdoidal suture.

5. **Occipital Bone**

The occipital bone forms the posterior part of the upper skull. It is readily visible from an inferior aspect, which is looking up at the bottom of the skull.

B. **Sutures**

Most of the skull's joints are essentially immovable joints called sutures. Extremely flexible and incomplete during birth, as the individual develops the sutures become more rigid.

1. **Sagittal**

The suture between the parietal bones.

2. **Coronal**

This suture follows an anterior coronal plane and is the suture between the frontal and parietal bones.

3. **Bregma**

The bregma is the intersection of the sagittal and coronal sutures.

4. **Lambdoidal**

The lambdoidal suture is at the intersection of the occipital and parietal bones. It looks somewhat like the Greek letter lambda or like an inverted "Y."

5. **Pterion (Squamosal)**

The squamosal suture is at the intersection of the frontal, sphenoid, parietal, and temporal bones. It has an "H" shape.

IV.   **Inferior Aspect of the Cranium**

A.   **Anterior Section**

The anterior section of the inferior skull is lower than the other sections. It consists of the upper dental arch and the palate. It is the bony foundation for the roof of the mouth.

1.   **Hard Palate**

The bony foundation of the hard palate is formed by the paired maxillae and palatine bones. This part of the vocal tract is extremely important for the articulation of consonants. All dental, alveolar, postalveolar, and palatal consonants are formed by juxtaposition of the tongue with this part of the skull. Palatal speech sounds include the ones we associate with the written letter "Y" or the phoneme /j/. However, postalveolar palatal contact is observed in a host of other speech sounds formed by bringing the tongue in contact with, or nearly with, the palate.

a.   *Maxillae:* The paired maxillae are complex bones that form most of the hard palate. Outside the oral cavity, they are facial bones.

(1)   *Palatine Processes:* The anterior portion (3/4) of the hard palate is formed by the palatine processes of the maxillae. These processes fuse in the middle during fetal development, moving inferiorly from a nearly vertical position to meet in the sagittal plane of the oral cavity. The fusion is called the median palatine suture. Failure of these processes to fuse is called a cleft palate, or maxillary cleft. There are several important landmarks of the hard palate.

(2)   *Superior Alveolar Processes:* The upper teeth are rooted in these portions of the maxillae (see alveolar ridge).

(3)   *Incisive Fossa:* This landmark separates the palate from the prepalate where the upper incisors grow. It is the hole through which arteries (sphenopalatine) and nerves (nasopalatine) pass.

b.   *Palatine Bone:* These bones have two sections: a perpendicular section and a horizontal section. The horizontal sections form the posterior part of the hard palate. They also form the inferior portions of the choanae. A small superior spine on each horizontal process also form the inferior parts of the posterior nasal septum. The rest of the inferior part of the nasal septum is formed by the vomer.

c. **Superior Teeth:** Phonemes requiring articulation with the teeth are called dental. In English they are all fricatives and include the sounds we associate with the sound "th" and the written letters "f" and "v." The lips articulate with the teeth for /f/ and /v/ and the tongue articulates with the teeth for /θ/ and /ð/.

(1) **Incisors:** The upper incisors are the teeth essential to speech articulation. There are four incisors: two central and two lateral. Only one upper incisor is necessary for dental phoneme production.

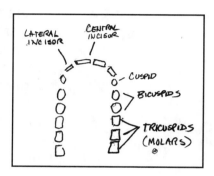

(2) **Cuspids:** The other teeth in the superior alveolus are not essential to normal speech articulation, but are important in mastication. Lateral to the incisors are the cuspids. The cuspids are sometimes called the canines or eyeteeth.

(3) **Bicuspids:** Next are the bicuspids, then the molars.

(4) **Molars:** Next to the bicuspids are the molars. The third molars are sometimes called the wisdom teeth. They erupt in early adulthood and are not part of the deciduous dentition.

2. **Growth and Development of Teeth**

a. **Teeth Eruption:** The deciduous upper incisors usually erupt by 8 to 10 months of age. The deciduous teeth are shed after the first molars erupt (6th year). This allows for the mastication of food while the anterior dentition is shed. Permanent incisors erupt in the 7th (central) and 8th (lateral) years.

b. **Anomalies of Occlusion:** The alveoli are remarkably flexible and the teeth may shift around in both bony arches during life. This shifting may cause anomalies in the way the upper teeth articulate with the lower teeth (occlusion). Anomalies in occlusion may affect mastication and speech articulation.

(1)   *Axiversion:* Tilting out of line in reference to the axis of the body.

(a)   **Distoversion:** Tilted toward the lips.

(b)   **Mesioversion:** Tilted toward the middle of the oral cavity.

(2)   *Infraversion:* Tooth not erupted to reach the line of occlusion.

(3)   *Supraversion:* Tooth has grown too far and protrudes into the line of occlusion.

(4)   *Torsiversion:* Twisted tooth (on its long axis).

B.   **Middle Section of the Skull**

The middle section of the inferior skull is most notable as the roof of the nasopharynx. It is formed by the sphenoid and occipital bones.

1.   **Nasopharynx**

The nasopharynx is the location of the upper portion of the pharynx. The nasopharynx extends from the choanae (pronounced "ko ANN ay") to the plane of the hard palate (palatal processes of the maxillae). The superior and posterior skeleton of the nasopharynx is formed by the sphenoid bone and the occipital bone. This is the roof of the nasopharynx. The inferior and anterior parts are formed by the bones that make up the palate and the posterior part of the nasal cavity.

2.   **Sphenoid Bone**

The front part of the middle section of the inferior skull is mainly formed by the body of the sphenoid bone. The sphenoid bone is irregularly shaped. Anatomists see it as having two sets of batlike wings. Some parts of the sphenoid bone are important for speech.

a.   *Pterygoid Plates:* The lateral and medial pterygoid plates are central structures of the area between the greater wings of the sphenoid bone. These parts of the sphenoid bone are points of attachment for pharyngeal muscles. They project down into the nasopharynx.

(1) *Pterygoid muscles:* The pterygoid muscles draw the mandible toward the sphenoid bone. Two pairs of pterygoid muscles arise from the lateral pterygoid plates and the surrounding palatine and maxilla bones. They insert on the interior surface of the mandible near the angle or farther up its ramus. Because there are two pairs, a variety of combinations of muscular contractions can allow the mandible to perform a circular movement. Speech pathologists like to call this movement a "rotary chew."

(2) *Tensor Veli Palatini:* The tensor veli palatini is part of the palatal elevation mechanism. It pulls the velum upward, and tenses it during speech and swallowing. Its name means "muscle that tenses the soft palate." This muscle originates on the inferior sphenoid bone anterior to its articulation with the temporal bone in the area known to anatomists as the sphenopetrosal fissure. Also, there are some origin fibers attached to the spine of the sphenoid bone and to the cartilaginous portion of the auditory eustachian tubes. The tendon of the tensor veli palatini winds around the hamulus of the medial pterygoid plate and inserts into the palatal aponeurosis. This pair of muscles tenses the velum during velar closure. It also helps equalize tympanic air pressure by mechanically opening the auditory tubes.

3. **Occipital Bone**

The occipital bone forms the posterior, and most of the basal part of the inferior cranium. The most anterior part of the occipital bone forms the pharyngeal tubercle, just in front of the foramen magnum. The pharyngeal aponeurosis (the fibrous portion of the pharynx above the superior constrictor), attaches to the pharyngeal tubercle of the occipital bone. This bony attachment allows the superior pharyngeal constrictor to alter the tension and dimensions of the nasopharynx and may provide posterior support for the velopharyngeal sphincter. Therefore, the occipital bone plays a role in changing the shape of in the resonating chamber and hence affects voice quality.

C.   **Posterior Section of the Inferior Skull**

1.   **Occipital Bone**

a.   ***Foramen Magnum:*** The foramen magnum is the largest hole in the inferior skull. In fact, its name means "big hole." Several important structures pass through the foramen magnum.

b.   ***Occipital Condyles:*** On either side, and slightly posterior to the foramen magnum, are the smooth occipital condyles. The occipital condyles are the points of articulation for the first cervical vertebra (C-1). It does not move much. It is called the atlas because it holds up the globe.

c.   ***Hypoglossal Canals:*** The hypoglossal canals are just inside lateral areas of foramen magnum. Through these canals pass the hypoglossal nerves, one on each side. These cranial nerves provide motor innervation to the tongue.

2.   **Temporal Bones**

a.   ***Squamous Portions:*** The temporal bones are visible from the inferior and lateral aspects of the skull. The squamous (flat) processes are most visible from the lateral aspect. This is the part called the "temple."

b.   ***Petrous Portions:*** The petrous portions are internal. Petrous means "rocklike." This part is located mostly inside the cranial cavity. In the petrous portions the following structures are found: auditory meatuses and bony labyrinths.

(1)   ***Auditory Meatuses:*** The external auditory meatuses are also known as the ear canals. The internal auditory meatuses are passages for the facial and vestibulocochlear nerves as well as the internal auditory arteries to pass into the cranium.

(2)   ***Bony Labyrinths:*** The bony labyrinths are a series of tunnels bored out of the petrous portions of the temporal bones. The inner ears and the balance (vestibular) mechanism are contained in these tunnels.

(3)   *Levator Veli Palatini:* The other palatal elevator is levator veli palatini; the name means "lifter of the soft palate." It arises or originates from the cartilaginous portion of the auditory eustachian tube and petrous portion of the temporal bone to insert in the palatal aponeurosis. An aponeurosis is a sheet of connective tissue. This connective tissue is in the middle of the velar muscles and allows the fibers of one levator veli palatini muscle to connect with the fibers of the one from the other side. When the levator veli palatini contracts it pulls the velum up, toward the sphenoid bone. It acts in concert with the tensor veli palatini to help close the velopharyngeal sphincter and uncouple the nasal cavity.

c.   *Mastoid Processes:* The mastoid processes are located just below and posterior to the external ears (pinnae). They are built of porous bone. Because there is a direct bony connection to the membranes of the inner ear, audiologists place bone vibrators here to see if the cochleae in the inner ears can pick up sound better when the bones are vibrated than they can when the sound is conducted by air. If so, this is an indication of a conductive hearing disorder. The spleniuscapitus, longissimus capitus, and sternocleidomastoid muscles insert at the mastoid process. The posterior belly of the diagastric muscle also inserts at the mastoid process.

d.   *Styloid Processes:* The styloid processes can be seen from the inferior aspect. These are shaped like pencils and are located deep in the opening of the external auditory meatuses. They point almost directly to the posterior tongue. The stylohyoid, stylopharyngeus, and styloglossus muscles attach here. The stylohyoid and stylopharyngeus muscles pull up the larynx (superiorly) during deglutition. You can feel (palpate) it by performing a dry swallow. This is a remarkable observation and one part of the swallowing evaluation. If the clinician cannot palpate the superior excursion of the laryngeal prominence during a dry swallow, it is a good clue that a swallowing pathology may exist.

e.   *Jugular Foramina:* The jugular foramina are lateral to the foramen magnum. Several important structures pass through these foramina, including the internal jugular veins and the glossopharyngeal, vagus, and the accessory nerves.

(1)   *Internal Jugular Veins:* The internal jugular veins return blood from the brain to the heart and lungs.

(2)   *Glossopharyngeal Nerves:* The glossopharyngeal nerve (IX) provides motor innervation to some muscles of deglutition and sensory (taste and touch) innervation to the posterior one-third of the tongue. Innervation means to provide nervous system connection and function.

(3)   *Vagus Nerves:* The vagus nerves (X) have fibers from accessory nerves that supply motor impulses to the larynx, pharyngeal constrictors, and muscles of palatal elevation. The vagus nerve (X) gives sensory innervation to the pharynx and motor impulses to the smooth muscles of the pharynx. Examples of smooth pharyngeal muscles are those in the carotid arteries. These involuntary muscles modify the blood flow to the brain as needed.

(4)   *Accessory Nerves:* The accessory nerves convey motor impulses to palatal elevators. Aberrant fibers go along with the vagus nerve (X) to the larynx and pharyngeal muscles. They also provide sensory innervation to the velum and oropharynx.

f.   *Carotid Canals:* The carotid canals are also located in the temporal bones. Through them course the following:

(1)   *Internal Carotid Arteries:* The internal carotid arteries supply blood to the brain.

(2)   *Sympathetic Plexuses:* Sympathetic plexuses are the main autonomic trunks providing involuntary control of the organs and other body parts to keep the systems running smoothly without our conscious input.

V.   **Anterior Aspect of the Skull**

A.   **The Face**

1.   **Importance in Communication**
The face has importance in communication through both auditory (speech and hearing) and visual (gesturing and visual) modalities.

a.   ***Speech***

- For the auditory modality of communication, we use the facial muscles to form several speech sounds. These include the labial sounds and the rounded vowels. Labial sounds are those we associate with the written letters "p," "b," "m," "w" (or wh), "f", and "V." The first four are formed with action of both the upper and lower lips, so they are called bilabial. The last two are formed by moving the lower lip against the upper teeth, so they are called labiodental.

- Lip rounding is done by tightening the lips and forming an "O" shaped hole (aperture) at the oral opening. The hole may be loose or tight, depending upon the needs of the speaker. Perhaps the tightest rounding happens when we make the vowel /u/. The loosest might be when we say /ɒ/. In between, there are /o/, and /ɔ/.

- Rounding makes the vocal tract slightly longer and adds a little more acoustic change at the lips. This acoustic change is called radiation impedance. Some other speech sounds, such as the /r/ and the /ʃ/ may also be accompanied by some lip rounding, depending upon the speaker.

b.   ***Facial Expression***

We use the muscles of facial expression to enhance our spoken communication with visual redundancy. This helps our listener understand what we have said. However, the listener is not the only one helped by the movements of the facial muscles. The speaker also receives feedback from the listener by watching his or her muscles of facial expression. We also use facial expression as a modality by itself. The eyes are located in the anterior aspect of the skull and we use them for expression, orientation, attention, and reading. Deaf signers also use facial expression to convey grammatical information.

2.   **Bones of the Face**

a.   ***Frontal Bone:*** The frontal bones are paired at birth and fuse during childhood. By the time an individual is 10 years old, the paired frontal bones have become fused to form a single bone. The front part of the calvaria and the majority of the orbits are formed by the frontal bone.

b. **Maxillae:** The paired maxillae form the superior alveolus from which the superior incisors erupt. These are important to speech articulation, as at least one incisor is required for production of dental speech sounds.

c. **Zygomatic Bones:** The zygomatic bones form the foundations of the cheeks. They articulate with the frontal bones and with the zygomatic processes of the temporal bones.

d. **Nasal Bones:** The tiny nasal bones form the bridge of the nose.

e. **Mandible:** Even though the mandible is not a proper part of the cranium, it is an essential part of the lower facial skeleton.

3. **Landmarks of the Face**

a. **Frontal Eminences:** There are two poorly defined frontal eminences located just above each orbit. These are little round knobs, more visible as facial features on some individuals than on others.

b. **Orbits:** The orbits are two of the cavities of the skull. The twin orbits house the eyes and are important for orientation and facial expression. The eyes are important for reading and writing, another form of communication.

c. **Nose:** The nose is the visible cover of the nasal cavity, the third of four important skull cavities discussed in this lecture. The nose and nasal cavity are important for speech purposes. They provide an alternate resonating cavity for the sounds made by the vocal tract, as well as an alternate air vent. English has three nasal speech sounds. They are the sounds we associate with the written letters: "m," "n," and "-ing." Several parts of the nose are important in evaluation of the peripheral speech mechanism.

(1) **Nares:** The outer (distal) margins of the nasal passages. The nares may be distorted by congenital or adventitious events. Such distortion may affect speech resonance.

(2)   *Nasal Septum:* The wall separating the nasal passages. A deviated nasal septum may result in hyponasal speech.

d.   *Philtrum:* The groove in the skin located below the nasal septum and extending inferiorly to meet the upper lip is called the philtrum. It is formed during fetal development by the fusion of the medial nasal and the maxillary processes.

VI.   Lateral Aspect of the Skull

A.   Bones

1.   Frontal Bone

We only see the side of the frontal bone from the lateral aspect. Looking from the side, we can see its articulation with the parietal and sphenoid bones, as well as with the zygomatic, nasal, lacrimal bones, and the maxilla.

2.   Parietal Bone

Only one of the paired parietal bones is visible. It articulates with the frontal, temporal, sphenoid, and occipital bones. Between the two parietal bones at the top of the skull is the sagittal suture.

3.   Sphenoid Bone

The greater wing of the sphenoid bone is most visible from the lateral aspect, but we can also see a portion of it in the orbit.

4.   Temporal Bone

The ear is housed entirely in the substance of the temporal bone. From the lateral viewpoint, we can see the bony portion of the external auditory meatus. Just inferior to the external auditory meatus is the pointy styloid process, and posterior to that is the mastoid process. Above the external auditory meatus is the flat squamous portion of the temporal bone. The temporal bone articulates with the zygomatic bones at its zygomatic process. It also articulates with other calvaria, including the frontal, sphenoid, parietal, and occipital bones.

a.   *External Auditory Meatus:* From the lateral aspect, we can see the proximal two-thirds of the external auditory meatus. The distal one-third is formed of elastic cartilage. This is significant because the flexible nature of the cartilage makes it possible to insert earplugs for protection or hearing aid ear molds for amplification.

b.   ***Mastoid Process:*** Immediately posterior to the external auditory meatus is a well-defined eminence called the mastoid process. It serves as a convenient location for placement of a transducer for assessment of bone conduction hearing thresholds.

c.   ***Styloid Process:*** The styloid process is a thin temporal bone process, projecting inferiorly and anteriorly below the external auditory meatus. The styloid process is the origin of three important muscles: styloglossus, stylo-hyoid, and stylopharyngeus.

5.   **Occipital Bone**

The occipital bone, the posterior portion of the calvaria, articulates with six other bones: the two parietal bones, the two temporal bones, the sphenoid, and the cervical atlas.

B.   Articulations

1.   **Temporo-Zygomatic**

You can see the zygomatic bones from the lateral aspect. They articulate with the temporal bones, the frontal bones, and the maxillae. Interestingly, the part of the temporal bone that articulates with the zygomatic bone is called the zygomatic process. The portion of the zygomatic bone that articulates with the temporal bone is called the temporal process.

2.   **Pterion**

The pterion can be described roughly as an "H"-shaped intersection of calvaria. It is the intersection of the frontal, parietal, sphenoid, and temporal bones.

VII.   The Mandible

The mandible articulates with the temporal bone at the temporomandibular joint. The mandible moves very little in normal speech. It does have importance in the production of speech. The mandible must be elevated for production of most consonants and most close or mid vowels.

A.   Importance in Speech

1.   **Tongue Elevation**

Mandibular elevation is required to bring the tongue within reach of the oral roof to form palatal, alveolar, labial, and dental phonemes. It is also required to form close vowels, like /i/ and /u/, and rhotic vowels (vowels with an /ɝ/ sound, as in earth).

2. **Opening of the Oral Cavity**

Open vowels are often produced with a more open oral aperture. Greater loudness can be achieved with a more open cavity. This is most important for public speakers and for singers.

3. **Point of Attachment for Muscles of Speech Articulation**

   a. *Muscles That Insert on the Interior Aspect of Mandible*

      (1) *Genioglossus:* The paired genioglossus muscles are the largest of the tongue muscles. It is fan-shaped and forms the majority of the tongue body. This muscle originates from the mental spine of mandible (interior, at the chin) and inserts into the tongue from tip to root. Some of the fibers insert into the hyoid bone. When the genioglossus muscles contract, the tongue sticks out.

      (2) *Mylohyoid:* A paired muscle, the mylohyoid forms the muscular floor of the anterior mouth. It attaches laterally to the anterior four-fifths of a slightly raised line on the interior aspect of the mandible, called the mylohyoid line. In its posterior middle section the mylohyoid attaches to the hyoid bone corpus. It has a median raphe running along its antero-posterior length, to which the opposing pairs are attached along the remainder of its middle.

      (3) *Superior pharyngeal constrictor:* This muscle originates at several locations. These attachments are to the most lower part of inferior border of the medial pterygoid plate, to the pterygomandibular raphe, and to the mandible, at a location posterior to the last molar. The superior pharyngeal constrictor inserts into the pharyngeal tubercle of occipital bone and the median raphe of pharynx.

      (4) *Lateral pterygoid:* This muscle has two heads. One originates from the lateral aspect of lateral pterygoid plate, and the other originates from the infratemporal surface of the greater sphenoid wing. The two bellies insert into the neck of the mandible and into the capsule of the temporomandibular joint.

      (5) *Medial pterygoid:* This muscle originates at the medial aspect of the lateral pterygoid plate and at

the posterior surface of the maxilla and palatine bones. It inserts into the medial aspect of the mandible near its angle. The medial and lateral pterygoids draw the mandible forward and side-to-side to produce the grinding action of the "rotary chew."

b. ***Muscles That Attach to the External Aspect of the Mandible***

(1) *Masseter:* This muscle originates at the lower border and the deep aspect of the zygomatic arch. It inserts into the wide area of the lateral aspect of the ramus and coronoid process of the mandible.

(2) *Temporalis:* This muscle originates on the surface of the lateral skull (parietal and temporal bones) and inserts into the tip and medial aspect of the coronoid process, as well as the anterior margin and medial aspect of the mandibular ramus.

(3) *Buccinator:* The buccinator inserts into the fibers of the orbicularis oris and the depressor anguli oris muscles from the alveolar processes of mandible and maxilla and the pterygomandibular raphe.

(4) ***Depressor labii inferioris and depressor labii anguli oris:*** These muscles lower the inferior lip. They originate on a line at the inferior border of the mandibular body on either side of the mental symphysis and insert into the fibers of the orbicularis oris and superficial fascia.

(5) *Platysma:* This muscle arises in the fascia inferior to clavicles and inserts at the lower border of the mandible and facial muscles.

B.   Importance in Deglutition

Mandibular movement is essential to normal mastication and, thus, normal deglutition. Mastication is the process of grinding a bolus of food between the teeth to prepare it for digestion. Some call this stage of swallowing the oral preparatory stage. After the oral preparatory stage, some authorities describe an oral stage during which the bolus is transferred to the pharynx. Others combine the preparatory and transfer stages into a single oral stage.

1. **Opening of the Oral Cavity**

   The mandible is depressed to admit food into the oral cavity. The bigger the piece of food, the more the mandible must be depressed. The muscles that help lower the mandible are the mylohyoid and the anterior belly of the digastric muscles. Once the food is placed in the mouth, the mandible is elevated, the lips seal the oral cavity, and the buccinator works with the tongue and lips to push food back into the oral cavity for processing.

2. **Mastication**

   Mastication involves a vertical chew and a rotary chew. The masseter and temporalis muscles accomplish the vertical chew, while the pterygoid muscles accomplish the rotary chew. One may consider the tongue an organ of mastication, as it helps keep the bolus between the teeth. In that case, the genioglossus and mylohyoid muscles are included. These muscles attach to the mandible.

C. **Structure of the Mandible**

   1. **Corpus**

      The U-shaped part of the mandible is the corpus. This is the "U"-shaped part.

      a. ***Mental Symphysis and Protuberance:*** At the anterior extent of the corpus is a prominence. Here the two sides of the mandible fuse in utero, and the fusion appears to continue postpartum, as cartilage in this site turns into bone. This protuberance is called the mental symphysis. A symphysis is a place where two structures have fused. The mental symphysis is the underlying structure of the chin.

      b. ***Inferior Alveolar Arch:*** Not much. We can speak quite well without our bottom teeth. Speech might sound a little unusual, but intelligibility will not suffer.

   2. **Ramus**

      This is the more vertical, flat portion of the mandible that projects superiorly to articulate with the temporal bone at the temporomandibular joint (TMJ).

      a. ***Condylar Process:*** The condylar processes articulate with the temporal bones at the mandibular fossae. The name of this process comes from the word condyle, which is a smooth part of a bone especially made for articulation.

b.   ***Temporomandibular Joint:*** The temporomandibular joint is a synovial joint. It tolerates a great deal of force, especially during mastication.

   (1)   ***Muscles of Mandibular Elevation:*** The muscles of mandibular elevation include the temporalis, masseter, and pterygoids.

   (2)   ***Muscles of Mandibular Rotation and Protrusion:*** The muscles of mandibular rotation include the medial and lateral pterygoids.

   (3)   ***Muscles of Mandibular Depression:*** Depression of the mandible occurs with contraction of the diagastric, mylohyoid, geniohyoid, and hyoglossus muscles.

c.   ***Coronoid Process:*** The coronoid process of the mandible is an elevated portion just anterior to the condylar process. This is where the temporalis muscle attaches.

d.   ***Angle of the Mandible:*** The angle decreases with the development of dentition and it increases with the loss of dentition. Thus, the mandibles of infants and edentulous adults are relatively flat when compared to those of individuals having complete sets of teeth.

VIII.   **The Speech Articulators**

   A.   **Overview**

      1.   **Form**

         a.   **Fixed Articulators**

         The fixed articulators include structures that are part of the maxilla and the palatine bone. Thus, the fixed articulators include the superior dentition, alveolar ridge, and "hard" palate (palatine processes of the maxilla and lateral process of palatine bone).

(1) *Upper Incisors:* There are four upper incisors, and these are used in the production of dental speech sounds. All the dental speech sounds are fricatives and involve either the articulation of the lower lip with the teeth or the articulation of the tongue with the teeth. The dental sounds are the ones we associate with the written letters "f," "v," and "th."

(2) *Superior Alveolar Ridge:* The superior alveolar ridge is the elevated lump of tissue behind the front teeth. The term "alveolar" refers to the open sockets from which the upper teeth erupt. The tongue articulates against this ridge for production of speech sounds called alveolar. The tongue elevates to produce these sounds, which we associate with the letters "t," "d," "n," "s," "z," and "l."

(3) *Hard Palate (Maxillae):* The tongue also elevates to produce the post alveolar and palatal sounds. We associate the palatal sounds with the written letters/sounds /j/, /r/, /ʃ/, and /ʒ/, /tʃ/, and /dʒ/. Plosive and nasal consonants can be articulated at the post alveolar place without creating phonemic contrast.

b. **Mobile Articulators**

The mobile articulators move in relationship to the fixed ones. Inside the mouth, mobile articulators would include the tongue and the velum. Other mobile articulators that are not specifically inside the oral cavity are the lips, mandible, glottis, and pharyngeal walls.

(1) *Lips:* Lips create what are called the labial consonants, including the sounds we associate with the written letters "p," "b," "m," "w," "f," and "v." The muscle surrounding the lips contracts to produce "rounded" vowels.

(2) *Mandible:* The mandible must be elevated to produce almost all the speech sounds. Glottal sounds and open back vowels can be articulated with a depressed mandible.

(3) *Soft Palate (Velum):* This is the soft tissue in the posterior of the oral cavity. If you look into a mirror,

you can easily see it. The velum drops down during articulation of nasal consonants and elevates to seal off the nasal cavity from the vocal tract during the production of all other sounds. Nasal sounds are associated with the letters "m," "n," and the suffix "-ing." The back of the tongue is elevated to contact the velum during production of the speech sounds we associate with the letters "k," "g," and the suffix "-ing."

(4) *Tongue:* This highly flexible organ can change the shape of the vocal tract in many ways. It is active in the production of almost all speech sounds. The only American English speech sounds the tongue is not involved in making are the ones we associate with the letters "p," "b," "m," "f," "v," and "h."

(5) *Pharyngeal Walls:* The pharyngeal walls are in constant motion during speech. Their actions change the shape and resonating characteristics of the vocal tract.

(6) *Larynx:* The larynx not only produces the sound of the voice, important in all but a few speech sounds, it also creates the sounds we associate with the letter "h," and a glottal sound that one could argue starts all isolated vowel sounds.

2. **Function in Speech**

   a. *Modulation of Airflow for Obstruent Consonant Articulation*

   The modification of airflow creates the plosive and fricative sources and routes the airflow through the oral or nasal cavities.

   b. *Alteration of Resonance for Vowel and Approximant Articulation*

   Resonance is an essential aspect of discrimination for all phonemes. When the cavity of the vocal tract changes shape, its acoustic qualities change. Thus, a source, whether plosive, fricative, or phonatory will sound slightly different depending on the shape of the resonating cavity into which it is propagated. This is the listener's basis for speech sound discrimination.

c. **Formation of *Cul-de-Sac* for Nasal Articulation**

The speech articulators block the oral cavity at the bilabial "alveolar" and velar locations to vary the resonance of nasal consonants.

3. **Function in Deglutition**

The primary biological function of the oral cavity is to act as the entrance to the digestive tract. Thus, all the structures we use for speech articulation have some function in eating. The oral cavity is also a secondary passage for respiration in the event that the nose is not patent.

a. *Retention of Material in Oral Cavity*

The first function of the oral cavity in food and liquid intake is to admit and retain material for consumption. For this function the primary structures are the lips, velum, and tongue. Digestion begins in the oral cavity where powerful enzymes (ptyalin) contained in saliva help prepare food for digestion. Saliva also contains mucin which lubricates the inside of the digestive tract and helps material pass.

b. *Protection of Airway*

Because the oral cavity is an entrance to the airway, there is always a danger of material from the digestive tract entering the respiratory system (aspiration). If there are sensory or motor problems in the oral cavity or in the laryngopharyx affecting control and manipulation of the bolus, the patient may be at risk for aspiration. Aspiration is a serious health condition that could lead to death. In many settings, it is the SLP's role to assess the patient's ability to swallow safely. If there is a disorder, the SLP will determine whether strategies can be implemented that will eliminate the aspiration risk and increase the patient's chances of maintaining nutrition and hydration by oral feeding alone. If such strategies are possible, the SLP will work with the patient and caregivers to train them in what should be done to eliminate the risk of aspiration. Sometimes the risk cannot be eliminated. When this is the case, it is the SLP's role to notify the physician. Alternative nutrition and hydration (e.g., NG tube, PEG tube, etc.) may be required until the swallowing problem improves. The patency of the airway is the primary concern in dysphagia treatment.

c.   *Sealing of Oral Cavity for Pressure Change*

Efficient deglutition requires a seal of the anterior oral cavity. The structures that create for this seal are the lips and velum.

d.   *Mastication*

Mastication of the food bolus breaks down the large masses and helps mix them with the first digestive fluid. Structures involved in mastication include the mandible, teeth, palate, velum, tongue, and lips. Mastication requires a mobile tongue and a rotary chewing action to be most effective. The muscles of mastication elevate and move the mandible laterally.

e.   *Transfer of Bolus*

Food in the oral cavity is compacted into a mulched body called a bolus. Once the bolus is prepared for passage out of the oral cavity, the tongue, palate, and velum coordinate to move it posteriorly into the oropharynx.

B.   **Oral Speech Articulators in Detail**

1.   **Extraoral (Facial) Articulators**

a.   **Lips**

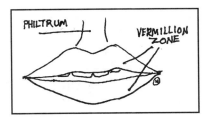

(1)   *Vermilion Zone*

This is the red fleshy area commonly referred to as the lips.

(2)   *Philtrum "Cupid's Bow"*

The superior curvature of the upper lip is a complex series of curves and recurves, much like a recurve bow used for archery. It has historically been a source of sexual attraction, and is thus called the cupid's bow.

(3)   *Effects of Lip Rounding*

When we round the lips during articulation of back vowels and some consonants, the anatomic result is to slightly lengthen the vocal tract. Added to this, in some cases, is the effect of radiation impedance. Radiation impedance is a soft friction that may be associated with sounds like "Oooo" and "wh." The lips also articulate in the production of labial consonants. The labial consonants are those we associate with the written letters: "p," "b," "m," "w," "wh," "f," and "v."

b.   **Muscles of Facial Expression**

(1)   *Sphincteric Muscles:* Sphincteric muscle fibers run in a circular direction around an opening. A sphincter is a muscular closure around an opening. On the face, the sphincters are the lips and the eyelids, which cover the oral cavity and the orbits, respectively. The sphincteric muscles are as follows:

(a)   *Orbicularis Oris:* This muscle encircles the oral opening. When its fibers contract, they tighten the lips. We have control over different portions of orbicularis oris fibers. To produce labiodental phonemes, only the inferior fibers of the orbicularis oris contract. Orbicularis oris also contracts for lip rounding.

(b)   *Orbicularis Oculi:* These muscle fibers encircle the orbits. Thus, they close the eyes, shielding them, allowing them to be cleaned and lubricated by tear secretions (lacrimation). A wink is created by contracting these muscle fibers and is a form of expression in some cultures, but it can have different meanings.

(2)   *Horizontal Muscles:* Horizontal muscle fibers all run roughly parallel to the transverse plane. All of them insert into the orbicularis oris muscle and act in opposition to it.

(a)   *Buccinator:* The buccinator is a thin muscle located in the cheek. It adds mechanical strength to the oral walls during sucking and can help draw the oral margins open.

(b)   *Risorius:* The risorius is another extremely thin muscle that runs from the facial tissue over the mandibular ramus and to the angles of the oral opening. When it contracts, it pulls the angles of the mouth toward the ears, making a grinning expression.

(3)   ***Angular Muscles:*** Angular muscles originate at various sites around the oral opening and insert into the fibers of the orbicularis oris. They act in opposition to the orbicularis oris, pulling the lips apart.

    (a)   ***Levator Labii Superiorus:*** The name means "lifter (like an elevator) of the upper lip," and that is the function of this muscle. It originates on the maxilla, below each orbit, and inserts into the orbicularis oris. When it contracts it draws the upper lip toward the eye.

    (b)   ***Levator Labii Superiorus Alaeque Nasi:*** The name of this muscle is the same as the one above, except that "alaeque nasi" means "beside the nose." It is medial to levator labii superiorus.

    (c)   ***Zygomaticus Major:*** Zygomaticus major and minor both originate on the zygomatic bones and insert into orbicularis oris. Contraction pulls the upper lip toward the zygomatic bone.

    (d)   ***Zygomaticus Minor:*** Zygomaticus major and minor both originate on the zygomatic bones and insert into orbicularis oris. Contraction pulls the upper lip toward the zygomatic bone.

    (e)   ***Depressor Labii Inferiorus:*** The name means "muscle that pulls the lower lip down (depresses it)." It originates in the mandible, near the chin, and draws the inferior lip in that direction.

(4)   ***Vertical Muscles:*** The vertical muscles also originate at points around the oral opening, but

their fibers take a more vertical course. They also oppose orbicularis oris.

(a) *Mentalis:* The mentalis originates on the mandible and inserts in the skin on the same area. Its action wrinkles the skin on the chin and causes the lower lip to protrude.

(b) *Depressor Anguli Oris:* The name means "muscle that pulls the angles of the mouth downward." It originates on the mandibular body and inserts into orbicularis oris.

(c) *Levator Anguli Oris:* This muscle's name means "muscle that lifts the oral angles." It orginates in the maxilla, inferior to the infraorbital foramen and inserts among the fibers of the orbicularis oris.

(5) *Parallel Muscles:* The parallel muscles are thin muscles running parallel to the upper and lower lips. They are called the incisivus labii superiorus and incisivus labii inferiorus. Both superior and inferior parallel muscles "purse" the lips to seal the oral cavity opening.

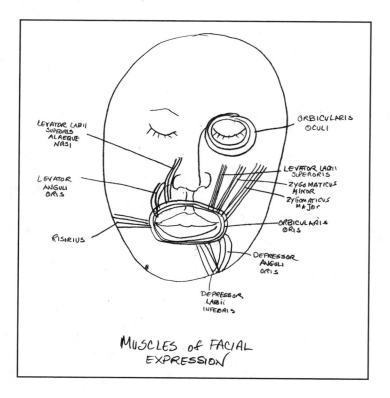

MUSCLES of FACIAL EXPRESSION

(a) *Incisivus Labii Superiorus:* This muscle originates on the maxilla just superior to the cuspid tooth and inserts among the orbicularis oris fibers.

(b) *Incisivus Labii Inferiorus:* This muscle originates on the mandible, just inferior to the lateral incisor and inserts among the orbicularis oris fibers.

c. **Function of Extraoral Articulators**

(1) *Labial Consonants:* Labial consonants consist of the speech sounds /p/, /b/, /m/, /w/, /ʍ/, /f/, and /v/.

(2) *Rounded Vowels:* Rounded vowels consist of speech sounds /ʊ/, /o/, /ɔ/, and /ɒ/. Lip rounding often accompanies articulation of /ʃ/, /ʒ/, and /r/.

(3) *Gestural Communication:* Imagine speaking without any facial expression; you have total paralysis of your facial muscles. Such a paralysis would not render you unable to communicate, but it would impose some difficulty for both speaker and listener. We rely heavily on our facial expressions to augment spoken communication. Perhaps this is made clear by the misunderstandings you may have during telephone or E-mail conversations.

(4) *Retention of Fluids:* An important role of the lips during fluid and food intake is to retain these in the oral cavity during mastication (chewing) and deglutition (swallowing). Many patients who have difficulty closing the oral opening also have trouble with speaking, chewing, and swallowing.

d. **Motor Innervation**

The muscles of facial expression receive their motor innervation through cranial nerve VII, also known as the facial nerve. Contraction of the facial muscles can occur voluntarily or involuntarily, depending on which parts of the brain and spinal cord are operating on the nerves of the face. When we smile or react to emotion, facial muscle contraction is involuntary. When we simply spread our lips the contraction is voluntary. Interestingly, the connections of the facial nerve to the voluntary motor tracts of the brain differ for the lower muscles and the upper muscles of facial expression. For voluntary contraction, the lower muscles receive upper motor innervation unilaterally, meaning that the nerves from one cerebral hemisphere connect only to those lower facial muscles on one side of the face. In this case (the case of the face), that side is the side opposite the cerebral hemisphere of origin. If the nerves in the right cerebral hemisphere are damaged, then the muscles of the lower face (below the orbits) will be paralyzed on the left side. The nerves that connect to the upper muscles of the face are innervated bilaterally, meaning that they have origins in both hemispheres. Thus, disease in one hemisphere will have no detectible clinical effect on the upper muscles (from the level of the orbits and superior) of facial expression.

f. **Sensory Innervation**

The trigeminal or fifth cranial nerve (cranial nerve V) conveys action potentials associated with pain, temperature, and gross or fine touch from the face to the brain. There are three branches of this nerve and each branch supplies a different area of the face. These sensation regions are called dermatomes.

2. **Intraoral Articulators**

a. **Roof of the Oral Cavity**

The "roof" of the oral cavity is founded on two bones: the palatine processes of the maxilla form the anterior three-quarters and the horizontal plates of the palatine bones form the posterior one-quarter. If there is a hole (fistula) in the "roof," the speaker will not be able to build up air pressure in the oral cavity. This would make it impossible to articulate speech sounds that require such air pressure build up in the oral cavity. Additionally, the permanent coupling of the nasal cavity to the vocal tract would create a constant nasal resonance, reducing the intelligibility of the speaker's production of non-nasal consonants and vowels.

(1) *Maxilla (Hard Palate)*

(a) *Tissue Type:* The hard palate is formed of mucous membrane covering the mucoperiosteum of the bones. Immediately posterior to the alveolar ridge, the examiner may observe corrugations on the surface. These corrugations are called rugae. Along the sagittal plane is a midline raphe. One may observe a torus palatinus, or thickening of periosteum and mucous membrane in the area of the intermaxillary suture (raphe). This thickening occurs in about 20% of individuals

(b) ***Superior Alveolar Ridge:*** The superior alveolar ridge is the seat of the superior dentition. For speech purposes,we are concerned mainly with the anterior section. Speech sounds formed by the tongue's articulation with this ridge.

(c) ***Upper Dental Arch:*** We have already discussed the upper dental arch. Remember, the most important teeth for speech purposes are the upper incisors. Speech sounds formed here by articulation with the anterior tongue or the inferior lip are called dental. Labiodental sounds are formed by articulation of the lower lip with the upper central incisors.

(2) ***Velum (Soft Palate)***

The soft palate, or velum, is composed grossly of epithelial tissue covering muscles. The muscles can draw the velum upward and back to articulate with the posterior and lateral pharyngeal walls, thus sealing the passage to the nasopharynx and directing air and acoustic energy through the oral cavity. They can also draw the velum down, coupling the nasopharynx to the vocal tract, or pulling the tongue upward.

(a) ***Uvula:*** The end of the velum drapes inferiorly with a free end known as the uvula.

(b) ***Velopharyngeal Sphincter:*** The anatomic structure that separates the nasopharynx from the rest of the vocal tract is known as the velopharyngeal sphincter because it is a rough ring of muscles and other soft tissue. This mechanism routes air and resonance through the oral or nasal cavities, depending on the requirements of the individual speech sounds.

i) **Muscles of the Velopharyngeal Sphincter**

a) *Tensor Veli Palatini:* This muscle originates on the inferior sphenoid bone anterior to its articulation with the temporal bone in the area known to anatomists as the sphenopetrosal fissure. Also, there are some origin fibers attached to the spine of the sphenoid bone and from the cartilaginous portion of the auditory (eustachian) tubes. The tendon of the tensor veli palatini winds around the hamulus of the medial pterygoid plate and inserts into the palatal aponeurosis. This pair of muscles contracts the velum during velar closure. It also helps equalize tympanic air pressure by mechanically opening the auditory tubes.

b) *Levator Veli Palatini:* This muscle originates at the petrous portion of the temporal bone and around the auditory tube. It inserts with its contralateral counterpart and together they lift the velum.

c) *Palatopharyngeus:* The palatopharyngeous muscle fibers have their ends in diverse locations, including the velum and pterygoid hamulus and auditory tube area of the pharynx. They insert into mucosa of pharynx, with some fibers attached to the thyroid cartilage. The palatopharyngeus forms the eminence of the posterior faucial arch. In function, they guide the bolus of food into pharynx. As elevators of the middle pharynx, they can also help to elevate the larynx.

d) *Palatoglossus:* The palato-glossus, as its name implies, is an extrinsic tongue muscle. Extrinsic means one end of the muscle is attached to the tongue, and the other end is attached somewhere else. In the case of the palatoglossus muscle, the "somewhere else" is the inferior surface of the palatine aponeurosis. The fibers insert into posterior sides of tongue. The paired palatoglossus muscles form the anterior faucial arch. When the paired palatoglossus muscles contract they can do one of two things: first, they can lift the back of the tongue up toward the velum; second, they can pull the velum down toward the back of the tongue. Pulling the back of the tongue toward the velum is used when we utter the sounds we associate with the written letters "k," "g," and the sound "ing." It is also useful in swallowing.

e) *Superior Pharyngeal Constrictor:* The superior pharyngeal sphincter is a circular muscle which attaches posteriorly to the occipital lobe and anteriorly to the sphenoid bone, mandible and connective tissue pterygomandibular raphe. It begins the squeezing action required for the pharyngeal stage of swallowing and helps tighten the velopharyngeal sphincter.

ii) **Function of the Velopharyngeal Sphincter**

When the velum is elevated, the oral cavity is disconnected from the nasal cavity. The resonance is described as oral. When the velopharyngeal sphincter is relaxed and allowed to open, the nasal cavity is coupled with the vocal tract, and the resonance is described as nasal. The velopharyngeal sphincter also closes during sucking and swallowing.

iii) **Motor Innervation**

Muscles cannot function without a motor nerve supply, and these muscles do not function well without nerves to convey touch sensations back to the central nervous system. Cranial nerves X and XI innervate the levator veli palatine and IX, X, and XI innervate palatoglossus and palatopharyngeus. The pharyngeal constrictors receive their motor innervation from a complex of the above cranial nerves plus some of the cervical spinal nerves. Cranial nerve V makes the tensor veli palatini contract. Sensory innervation is accomplished by branches of IX, X, and XI.

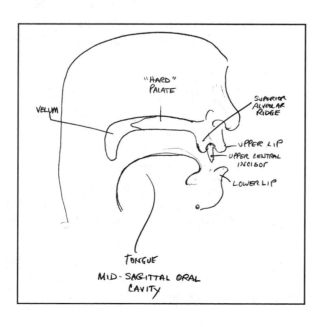

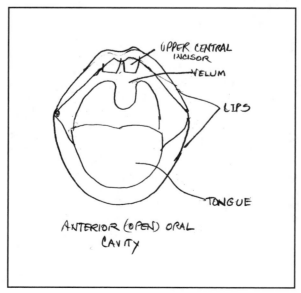

b.   **Floor of the Oral Cavity**

(1)   ***The Tongue***

The tongue is a highly mobile structure. Its great flexibility is essential for speech articulation. Movements of the tongue simultaneously alter the shape of the oral and pharyngeal cavities. The flexibility of the tongue enables the speaker to place obstructions in the oral cavity to impede the flow of air. These obstructions create the sounds associated with the obstruent consonants. Such sounds are the explosions of the plosives ("p," "b," etc.), and the hisses" of fricatives ("s," "z," etc.). Changing the shape of the oral cavity changes the way it and the rest of the vocal tract resonates. Listeners perceive changes in resonances with vowel and sonorant consonant changes.

(a)   **Gross Structure of the Tongue**

i)   ***Parts of the Tongue***

a)   *Apex:* The apex is the part of the tongue nearest the front teeth. Phoneticians sometimes call it the tip.

b)   *Dorsum:* This is the surface of the tongue extending from under the roof of mouth, where it may be referred to as the palatine part, to the oropharynx, where it is called the pharyngeal part. The palatine and pharyngeal parts are separated by a V-shaped sulcus, the sulcus terminalis.

c)   *Front:* The palatine dorsum is made up of the front (under the hard palate).

d)   *Back:* . . . and the back (under the velum).

e)   *Blade:* The part of the dorsum lying next to the superior alveolar ridge is referred to as the blade. The blade runs all around the sides of the tongue.

(f)   *Root:* The root is the extreme posterior part of the tongue. It is not used much in speech, but it is important because it is the part through which nerves, arteries, and veins run.

ii)   ***Tissue Type of the Tongue:*** The tongue is made up of muscle tissue covered with stratified squamous epithelium. The epithelium is marked by rows of small projections called papillae. These come in several shapes and contain taste organs among their epithelial cells. This epithelium is thin at the anterior two-thirds. Giving structure to the tongue, as well as serving as an attachment for the intertwined intrinsic musculature, is a fibrous skeleton called the corium. The main feature of the corium is a septum that divides the tongue into right and left halves.

iii)   ***Landmarks of the Tongue:*** There are several landmarks of the tongue. The anterior portion of the tongue is called the *tip*. The portion just below the alveolar ridge is the *blade*. Just below the hard palate lies what is known as the *front* of the tongue. Finally, the most posterior portion of the tongue which lies below the soft palate is called the back of the tongue.

iv)   ***Attachments of the Tongue:*** The tongue attaches anteriorly to the inside of the mandible at the mandibular symphysis, inferiorly to the hyoid bone, and posteriorly to the base of skull and the pharynx.

v)   ***Intrinsic Muscles of the Tongue:*** The intrinsic muscles of the tongue originate and insert within the body of the tongue, and compose most

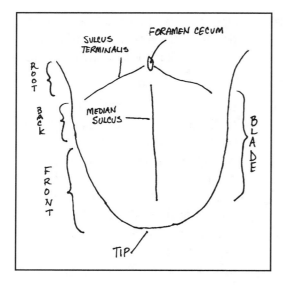

of the tongue mass. They are in four groups on either side of the septum and function to change the shape of the tongue. The intrinsic tongue muscles are named after the direction in which their fibers run: vertical, transverse, superior longitudinal, and inferior longitudinal.

a)   *Vertical muscles:* The vertical muscles, as their name suggests, span the superior-inferior dimension of the tongue. They originate and insert in the mucosa of the dorsum on the inferior surface, and their fibers pass through those of the superior and inferior longitudinal muscles (Saito & Itoh, 2003). Vertical muscle contractions flatten the blade of the tongue opposing the action of the transverse muscles.

b)   *Transverse muscles:* The transverse muscles originate at the fibrous septum and insert in the lateral mucosa, along the length of the tongue blade. Like the vertical muscles, the transverse muscle fibers penetrate the finer bundles of the longitudinal muscles as they cross through (Saito & Itoh, 2003). Transverse muscle contractions pull the lateral aspects of the tongue toward each other, shortening the distance between the sides. With full contraction of the transverse fibers the vertical dimension of the tongue's body increases. This contraction draws the lateral aspects of the lingual body medially, and pushes the tongue's dorsum closer to the palatal vault (essentially, thickening the tongue). This posture is appropriate for the palatal approximant, /j/. When contractions are limited to the upper fibers of the transverse muscle, the tongue's sides curl inward; in coordination with contractions of the superior longitudinal muscles, the blade and apex will be brought into contact with the lateral and anterior teeth. This lingual posture produces the proper oral cavity shape for dental-alveolar-postalveolar approximant, /r/.

c) *Longitudinal muscles:* The longitudinal muscle fibers run the length of the tongue's body, just beneath the epithelium on the superior surface (dorsum) and inferior surface, from root to tip. There are superior and inferior longitudinal muscles in the tongue.

d) *Superior longitudinal muscles:* Contractions of the superior longitudinal muscle curl the tongue's tip superiorly, bringing it into contact with the oral roof: the upper teeth, superior alveolar ridge and palate. This muscle is important for the production of dental and alveolar consonants.

e) *Inferior longitudinal muscles:* Contractions of the inferior longitudinal muscles curl the tip inferiorly, opposing the action of the superior longitudinal muscles.

vi)   ***Extrinsic Muscles of the Tongue:***
Like all extrinsic muscles, the extrinsic tongue muscles have their attachments outside the body of the tongue. Having an external attachment enables them to move the body of the tongue.

a)   *Genioglossus:* This paired muscle is the one you use to stick out your tongue. It forms most of the body of the tongue. Its anterior attachment is at the mental spine of the mandibular symphysis, or inside of the chin. Fibers run posteriorly and insert into the body of the tongue and into the hyoid bone. Contraction of genioglossus draws the tongue forward.

b)   *Styloglossus:* The styloglossus originates at the styloid process of the temporal bone and inserts into the posterior part of the tongue. Contraction of the styloglossus draws the body of the tongue backward, toward the styloid process. This movement is useful in swallowing.

c)   *Hyoglossus:* The hyoglossus muscles run from the sides of the tongue down to the greater horns of the hyoid bone. They can either draw the hyoid bone up, toward the tongue, or draw the sides of the tongue down, toward the hyoid bone.

d)   *Palatoglossus:* The muscular foundation of the anterior faucial arch, the palatoglossus originates on the inferior surface of the palatine aponeurosis. Its fibers insert into the posterior sides of the tongue. When the paired palatoglossus muscles contract, they can do either of two things; first, they can lift the back of the tongue up toward the velum; or they can pull the velum down toward the back of the tongue. Pulling the back of the tongue toward the velum is used when we utter the sounds we associate with the written letters "k," "g," and the sound "-ing." The function of this muscle is also important in swallowing.

vii) ***Motor Innervation of the Tongue:*** The intrinsic and extrinsic muscles of the tongue receive their motor innervation from cranial nerve XII, also called the hypoglossal nerve.

viii) ***Sensory Innervation of the Tongue:*** Sensory information coming from the tongue is generated by two kinds of stimuli. Somesthesis of tongue tissue is interpreted as touch temperature or pain, and changes in chemistry are interpreted as taste.

    a) ***Touch:*** Touch sensations arrive at the central nervous system via cranial nerve V if the stimuli are delivered from the anterior two-thirds of the tongue, and via cranial nerve IX from the posterior two-thirds.

    b) ***Taste:*** Taste sensations originating at the anterior two-thirds of the tongue are conveyed to the CNS via cranial nerve VII. Those from the posterior one-third travel via cranial nerve IX.

c. **Posterior Oral Cavity**

(1) ***Faucial Arches:*** Along the posterior sides of the oral cavity one can see two arches. These are the faucial arches. They are covered with the mucosal epithelium, but supported by two muscles: palato-glossus and palatopharyngeus.

(a) ***Palatoglossus:*** See above.

(b) ***Palatopharyngeus:*** See above.

(c) ***Tonsillar Fossa:*** Between the two arches is a triangular tonsillar fossa on either side. Here, if they have not been removed surgically, we will find parts of Waldeyer's ring—the faucial or palatine tonsils.

(2) ***Tonsils (Waldeyer's Ring):*** The lymphoidal tissues that make up Waldeyer's ring are the tonsils. There are three sets of tonsils. They are the palatine tonsils, the pharyngeal tonsils (adenoid tonsils), and the lingual tonsils.

(a) ***Palatine Tonsils:*** The palatine tonsils are located on the right and left, between the faucial arches.

(b) ***Pharyngeal (Adenoid):*** A single pharyngeal tonsil is located in the posterior pharynx, between the oropharynx and nasopharynx.

(c) ***Lingual:*** The lingual tonsil forms the superficial tissue of the tongue root.

(d) ***Functions:*** The tonsils help protect the entrance to the airway and digestive tract from bacterial infection. When they become overwhelmed, they swell and can become infected.

(e) ***Relevance to Speech Pathology:*** If the tonsils are removed, a procedure done frequently in the past, but not so often these days, a temporary combination of tissue insufficiency and incompetence may result. "Insufficiency" is the term applied when there is not sufficient tissue to form closure in the velopharyngeal sphincter. "Incompetence" applies when there is sufficient tissue, but the speaker is not using it efficiently ("competently"). In cases where the pharyngeal tonsil is removed, the removal of the lymphoidal tissue changes the dimensions of the oro/nasopharyngeal area, creating a temporary insufficiency. The speaker is accustomed to closing the velopharynx with the tissue present, and remains temporarily "Incompetent." Some speakers have difficulty compensating for the loss of the palatal tonsil. This insufficiency results in hypernasality. A short regime of speech therapy may help the speaker return to normal resonance, with an excellent prognosis for rapid recovery.

(3) *Posterior (Oro) Pharyngeal Wall:* The posterior pharyngeal wall moves inward to articulate with the velum for velopharyngeal sphincter functions. In normal people this movement is minimal. However, where a tissue insufficiency exists, such medial pharyngeal compensation may be encouraged therapeutically.

    (a) *Superior and Middle Pharyngeal Constrictors:* The superior and middle pharyngeal constrictors underlie the mucosa of the oropharynx.

    (b) *Passavant's Pad:* Passavant's pad is a small soft tissue eminence in the posterior pharyngeal wall. It may serve as an articulation point for the velum.

d. **Functions of Intraoral Articulators**

The intraoral articulators are all found inside the mouth. These structures play roles in formation of most of the phonemes of all languages. The intraoral articulators can be grouped into "fixed" and "mobile" categories. The fixed articulators are parts of the skull, and the mobile articulators move about in relationship to them. When the mobile articulators move in relationship to the fixed articulators, most often with accompanying phonation, a wide variety of sounds can be produced. Any sound we can create with the vocal tract is called a *phone*. Not all the sounds we can make with our vocal tracts are used in English. For instance, the bilabial trill, used by babies as they play with their lips, is not used in any English word. Similarly, there are sounds we use in English that aren't used in other languages. For instance, the sound we associate with the written letter, "r," is not used in Spanish or French. A sound, or really, a group of similar sounds, used in language to convey meaning, is called a phoneme. We say a phoneme is a group of similar sounds because each time a speaker targets that phoneme (e.g., /r/), it may come out a little different.

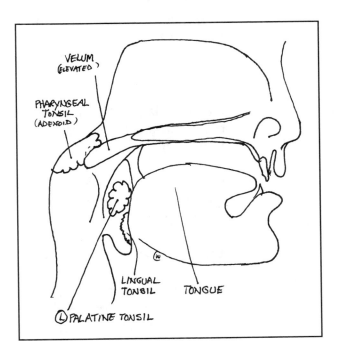

IX.   **Deglutition**

   A.   **Three Stages of Deglutition**

      1.   **Oral Stage (Voluntary)**

         a.   ***Preparation of the Bolus:*** The material to be consumed and assimilated (made part of the body) is broken down into a form that may be passed into the rest of the digestive tract. It is torn from its original position with the anterior teeth, the incisors, and ground up between the upper and lower posterior teeth. This process is called mastication. The chunk of food to be swallowed is called a "bolus." A vertical and rotary action accomplishes mastication best. During preparation, the first stage of chemical treatment commences. Food is mixed with saliva, which contains chemicals to break the complex food molecules down into less complex ones. Some consider this phase of the oral stage as a separate stage called the "oral preparatory" stage.

b. ***Elevation of Oral Floor:*** Elevation of the oral floor by the dorsum of the tongue begins the transfer of the bolus posteriorly toward the oropharynx.

c. ***Posterior Propulsion of Bolus:*** Following preparation of the food, the oral stage continues with the process of moving the food in a posterior direction, toward the oropharynx. The bolus is propelled posteriorly by combined action of the tongue, and to some extent the cheeks.

d. ***Constriction of Posterior Oral Cavity:*** At the right moment, the posterior oral cavity constricts by contraction of the faucial arches.

e. ***Closing of Velopharyngeal Sphincter:*** The velopharyngeal sphincter closes to prevent leakage into the nasopharynx.

2. **Pharyngeal Stage (Involuntary)**

a. ***Bolus Propulsion:*** The sequential constriction of the digestive trace propels swallowed material to be digested. This begins with the superior pharyngeal constrictor.

b. ***Approximation of Aryepiglottic Folds:*** During the pharyngeal stage, the aryepiglottic folds are approximated, sealing the laryngeal entrance.

c. ***Arytenoid Cartilages Drawn Superiorly and Anteriorly:*** The arytenoid cartilages are drawn superiorly and anteriorly during this action.

d. ***Elevation of Larynx and Articulation of Epiglottis:*** Simultaneously, the larynx is elevated and the epiglottis is drawn to a more horizontal position.

3. **Esophageal Stage (Involuntary)**

After this point, the bolus enters the esophagus and heads down into the stomach. There is not much a normal individual can do to control the bolus in the esophageal stage.

UNIT 6

THE NERVOUS SYSTEM

I.   **General Organization of the Human Nervous System**

- The human nervous system is organized into the peripheral and central systems. The distinction is for ease of study only, as each system is dependent on the other. In general, the peripheral system senses changes in the environment (internal or external) and conveys that information to the central system.

- Changes in the environment are called "stimuli." Examples of stimuli are changes in light (visual stimuli) or changes in acoustic energy (auditory stimuli). The central nervous system reacts to the input and responds by sending signals back to the peripheral system. Action is taken in response to environmental stimuli through the peripheral nervous system section.

- There is some anatomic and physiologic basis for the distinction among the peripheral and central systems. For example, the central system can be described in terms of specific structures. Also, there are differences in the nature of the support cells of the two systems. What's more, there are differences in how the systems recover from injury. The peripheral system tends to regenerate damaged neurons, while the central system has more redundancy.

A.   **Basic Structures**

1.   **The Neuron**

The neuron is the active functional unit of the nervous system. Neurons are distinguished by their abilities to convey changes in chemical polarity along their cell membranes and to deliver these changes to neighboring neurons.

a.   **Cell Body**

Each neuron is composed of a cell body, also called a "soma," or a "perikaryon," and one or more protoplasmic projection(s) called "neurites." There are two types of neurites: axons and dendrites.

b.   **Axon**

In general, axons conduct the action potentials away from the cell body.

c.   **Dendrite**

Dendrites conduct action potentials toward the cell body.

d.   **Synapses**

The synapse is the means by which neural impulses travel from one part of the cell body or from one neuron to another. One neuron connects with another by communicating the action potentials across the synaptic cleft (synapse).

2. **Glial Tissue**

The other type of tissue in the human nervous system is glial tissue. Glial cells support the neurons. This support includes holding the neurons in place as well as nourishing them. There are several types of glial cells. One type forms the framework to hold the neurons in place. Some insulate the axons, and others secrete a special fluid called cerebrospinal fluid. Still others play an important role in the removal and ingestion of degenerative debris or blood clots following hemorrhage. There is growing evidence that some glial cells are responsive to the same depolarizing stimuli that trigger responses in neurons, but their functions in action potential propagation are not yet clear.

B. **Central Nervous System**

1. **Brain**

The brain is the processor of the highest, most complex level of human nervous system activity. The more complex processing takes place at the thin outer layer of the brain. Gradually less complex activity takes place at more caudal locations. The brain is contained in the cranium and is divided from the spinal cord by a geographic (rather than functional) landmark: the foramen magnum. The foramen magnum is the opening at the base of the skull through which the spinal cord passes. The brain itself can be considered to consist of several distinct, but interacting, components.

a. **Cerebral Hemispheres**

The most advanced part of the brain is called the forebrain (prosencephalon). The forebrain is composed of two structurally and functionally similar halves called the cerebral hemispheres. Each hemisphere consists of an outer layer of cerebral cortex, an intermediate mass of white matter fibers, and an inner mass of gray matter fibers called the "basal nuclei" (basal ganglia).

(1) **Cerebral Cortex**

(a) *Location:* The covering of the cerebral hemispheres, like similar coverings of other organs, is called the cortex. The cerebral cortex is a thin (1.25–4.0 mm) covering of both cerebral hemispheres. It covers the outer and inner surfaces of the hemispheres.

(b) *General Function:* It is in the cerebral cortex that most of what we call "thinking" takes place. The cerebral cortex interprets and organizes stimuli from the peripheral nervous system, and formulates and organizes appropriate output.

(2) **Subcortical Structures**

(a) *Location:* Beneath the cortex lie several subcortical structures. They are not completely understood, but must function in concert in order for the organism to respond properly to environmental changes. There are several subcortical structures, including the basal ganglia and the thalamus.

(b) *General Function:* The basal nuclei function in a highly complex interactive manner, with multisynaptic neuronal projections and circuits. They seem to enhance the smooth execution of movement and probably play a larger, though subconscious, role in cognition. The thalamus is the relay center for all sensory input except smell. It also seems to play a role in affect.

b. **Brainstem**

(1) *Location:* The brainstem extends from the thalamus to the spinal cord and consists of three sections: midbrain, pons, and medulla. The midbrain (mesencephalon) is the most rostral part of the brainstem. Next is the pons and, finally, at the caudal end of the brainstem, is the medulla oblongata.

(2) *General Function:* The brainstem serves as the relay center for tracts of the spinal cord and the rest of the CNS. It integrates various CNS functions at an unconscious level (balance, reticular activation, ocular muscles, auditory localization). Nuclei (cell bodies) of most of the cranial nerves are located here, but these, of course, are not part of the brainstem. They are parts of the peripheral nervous system.

c. **Cerebellum**

(1) *Location:* Behind and below the cerebral hemispheres is the smaller cerebellum. It also has two hemispheres. The cerebellum overlies the brainstem and has special interaction with it and with the cerebral hemispheres. It is connected to the brainstem by three large fiber systems: the inferior, middle, and superior cerebellar peduncles. The cerebellum, like the midbrain, pons, and medulla, derived from the primitive esencephalon and rhombencephalon.

(2) *General Function:* The general function of the cerebellum is to coordinate action of antagonistic muscle groups. The cerebellum does not initiate motor activity, but coordinates it.

2. **Spinal Cord**

The spinal cord is the extension of the central nervous system beyond the skull. It is also called medulla spinalis.

a. *Location:* It extends from the level of the foramen magnum to that of the intervertebral space between the first and second lumbar vertebrae and is contained in the intervertebral canal of the spinal column. Do not get the spinal cord and the spinal column confused.

b. *General Function:* The spinal cord serves as the conduit for the major ascending and descending neural impulses. In the center of the cord is a gray core, shaped somewhat like a butterfly. This central core is surrounded by vertically coursing white fibers. This white area is composed of a number of separate bundles of nerves or axons called "tracts."

C. **Peripheral Nervous System**

The peripheral nervous system has two subdivisions: the cranial and spinal nerves and the autonomic nervous system.

1. **Spinal and Cranial Nerves**

a. **12 Cranial Nerves**

The cranial nerves are distinct in that most of them have their cell bodies in or near the brainstem. This means they supply central nervous system connections to the head and neck. Cranial nerve X, the vagus nerve, also supplies CNS connections to the thorax and abdomen. Besides their locations and the structures they innervate, another significant difference between cranial nerves and spinal nerves lies in their special sensory functions. The only afferents from spinal nerves are somesthetic, whereas cranial nerves convey impulses generated by visual, auditory, olfactory, and gustatory end organs, in addition to those of somesthesis. Cranial nerve axons run in a variety of directions, depending on their functions. Nerves that have their cell bodies aggregated (ganglia) near the foramen magnum have some rootlets emerging from the rostral end of the spinal cord. Each cranial nerve has a name and a number. The nerves are generally numbered from rostral to caudal. This means that cranial nerve I (one) is the most rostral and number XII (twelve) is the most caudal. Some anatomists consider the olfactory and optic nerves part of the central nervous system.

b. **31 Spinal Nerves**

The spinal nerves have their cell bodies in or near the spinal cord. There are 31 pairs of them. Like the cranial nerves, the spinal nerves also play roles in communication. Their most important one for speech is to allow expansion of the thoracic cavity in respiration. The spinal nerves also provide connections between the central nervous system and the extremities for their communicative functions.

2. Autonomic Nervous System

The autonomic nervous system (ANS) regulates the internal systems of the body to maintain optimum conditions for survival. It innervates smooth muscles (vascular, reproduction, respiratory, alimentary, glandular), cardiac muscles, and glands. The ANS has two main divisions: sympathetic and parasympathetic.

a. *Sympathetic Division:* The sympathetic division's primary function is to prepare the body for emergency action.

b. *Parasympathetic Division*: The parasympathetic division's primary function is to maintain regular bodily functions.

II.   **Central Nervous System**

A.   **The Brain in Detail**

1.   **Cerebral Hemispheres**

In the adult human being, the cerebral hemispheres are the largest part of the brain. They have evolved into highly complex structures that enable the individual to associate stimuli with great complexity. The hemispheres are almost mirror images of one another, and are functionally similar. They are separated by the longitudinal fissure.

a.   **Cerebral Cortex**

The cerebral cortex is a thin layer of gray (unmyelinated) tissue that coats the surface of the hemispheres. It varies in thickness from 1.25 to 4.0 millimeters. Because it developed at such a fast rate, it became wrinkled and is marked by elevations and depressions over its surface. The elevated areas are called gyri, and the depressed areas are called fissures or sulci. Some of these sulci or gyri are similar among different individuals, and have similar functions.

(1)   **Structure of the Cerebral Cortex**

The cortex is stratified. The layers are separated by thin bands of myelinated white matter running horizontally to connect the various surface regions of the brain. Vertically running fibers connect the layers to each other and to deeper parts of the brain. The surface of the cortex has been mapped by anatomists who have hypothesized and demonstrated specialty of functions to the different cells that compose the various regions. For example, the kind of neurons that compose the parts of the brain associated with reception of visual images are stratified differently from those associated with reception of auditory signals.

(a)   **Major Sulci of the Cerebral Cortex**

i)   *Longitudinal Fissure:* The longitudinal fissure separates the two cerebral hemispheres.

ii) *Lateral Sulcus (Fissure of Sylvius):* Looking at the brain from the side, the lateral sulcus is obvious.

iii) *Location of the Lateral Sulcus:* It runs posteriorly and superiorly between the temporal lobe, frontal, and parietal lobes.

iv) *Insula:* Deep to the lateral fissure is the insular cortex (or insula). It is also called the "Island of Reil." The function of the insular cortex is unclear at this time, but some physiologists believe it is associated with gustatory impulses. The insula is sometimes called the opercular cortex because the tissue of the temporal, frontal, and parietal lobes fold over it.

v) *Opercula:* The tissue of the temporal frontal and parietal lobes that folds over the insula is called the "opercula." The degree of coverage or folding over is called "operculization." Operculization is felt by some to be indicative of the degree of cortical development of growth. In the fetus, you can still see the insular cortex. In cases of arrested development, there is incomplete operculization, and the insula remains exposed.

vi) *Parallel Sulcus:* The parallel sulcus is parallel to the sylvian fissure. It is also called the superior temporal fissure and separates the superior temporal gyrus from the middle temporal gyrus.

(b) **Central Sulcus (Fissure of Rolando)**

Another very important cortical landmark is the central fissure.

i) *Location of the Central Sulcus:* The central sulcus separates the frontal and parietal lobes. It extends from the upper margins of the hemispheres to about the middle of the lateral sulcus, and is about 9 to 10 centimeters long.

ii) *Precentral and Postcentral:* Certain cerebral functions are described as "pre-" or "post-" central. Motor functions are "pre-" and sensory functions are "post-."

(c) **Major Gyri of the Cerebral Cortex**

i) *Precentral Gyrus:* The elevated area just anterior to the central fissure is called the "precentral gyrus." It is associated with motor functions and is called the "motor strip."

ii) *Postcentral Gyrus:* Just posterior to the central fissure is the postcentral gyrus. It is associated with tactile sensation and is sometimes called the "somesthetic cortex." Both the pre- and postcentral gyri are laid out in a somatotopic pattern. This means that their surfaces correspond roughly to the surface of the human body, beginning with the head at the most inferior end and finishing with the toes tucked down inside the longitudinal fissure.

iii) *Angular Gyrus:* At the end of the parallel sulcus lies the cortical center associated with coding written language. This is the angular gyrus, and it is part of Wernicke's area.

iv) *Supramarginal Gyrus:* At the upturned end of the lateral fissure lies the supramarginal gyrus. It is also part of Wernicke's area and is associated with decoding and encoding spoken language.

v) *Pars Triangularis:* Broca's area (pars triangularis) is found in the lower anterior area of the frontal lobe, but only in the dominant hemisphere. The neural pools here are associated with programming the sequential movements of speech.

(2) **General Functions of Areas of the Cerebral Cortex**

We associate certain functions to various parts of the cerebral cortex.

(a) *Sensory Cortex:* The sensory cortex is located in the postcentral gyrus.

(b) *Motor Cortex:* The motor cortex includes all of the precentral gyrus and the posterior portions of the frontal gyri.

(c) *Auditory Cortex:* The auditory cortex is found in the superior temporal gyrus.

(d) *Visual Cortex:* The visual cortex surrounds the calcarine sulcus.

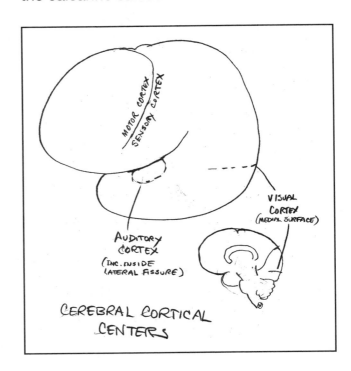

CEREBRAL CORTICAL CENTERS

2.   **General Hemispheric Functions**

a.   **Interhemispheric Differences**

The cerebral hemispheres function as whole entities, as does the entire central nervous system. However, there are certain functional differences between the left and the right hemispheres.

(1)   **Cerebral Dominance**

At first, the hemispheres appear to be identical. However, the dominant hemisphere is slightly heavier and slightly larger. This hemisphere also plays the major role in language formulation, analytic thought, and memory. The nondominant hemisphere appears to play a major role in thought, including such things as music, suprasegmentals, intuitive thinking, and so forth.

(a)   **Incidence of Left or Right Hemisphere Dominance:** The left hemisphere is dominant (i.e., damage results in significant language impairments) in 90% of right-handed people and 64% of left-handed people. The right hemisphere is dominant in 20% of left-handed people and in 60% of ambidextrous people. Both hemispheres are dominant in 30% of ambidextrous people (see Zemlin,W. [1998]. *Speech and Hearing Science: Anatomy and Physiology* [4th. ed., pp. 364–365]. Englewood Cliffs, NJ: Prentice-Hall).

(b)   **Relationship to Handedness:** Most people have dominant left hemispheres. However, because most people are also right handed does not mean that handedness is directly related to hemispheric dominance.

(2)   **Dominant Hemisphere Functions**

The dominant hemisphere is thought to play a major role in language formulation, analytic thought, and memory.

(3)   **Nondominant Hemisphere Functions**

The nondominant hemisphere appears to play the major role in holistic thinking: music, supraseg- mentals, and intuitive thinking.

b.   **Interhemispheric Communication**

There are four major connections between the cerebral hemispheres. The major bridge between the hemispheres is the corpus callosum. Smaller connections are the anterior commissure, the posterior commissure and the habenular commissure.

c.   **Intrahemispheric Communication**

Intrahemispheric communication pathways enable the integration of various cerebral functions. Remember, the whole system must act in concert. Intrahemispheric connections enable the functions of one hemisphere to coordinate. Short fibers connect adjacent convolutions, and long fibers connect more distant areas. There are three main long fiber bundles (fasciculi). The arcuate fasciculus is the major relay for language information from the posterior to the anterior parts of the brain. The unicate fasciculus connects the inferior frontal cortex (over the orbits) with the anterior temporal lobe. The cingulum connects areas of the frontal and parietal lobes with the temporal lobe and the hippocampus.

3.   **Lobes of the Cerebral Cortex**

The cerebral cortex can be divided into four lobes. The lobes are named after the bones of the calvaria under which they lie: frontal, parietal, temporal, and occipital. Bearing in mind that the brain functions best as a whole (in concert), physiologists have attributed functional roles to the lobes. These functions may be described as either primary or association.

a.   **Frontal Lobe**

(1)   **Location:** The frontal lobe lies beneath the frontal bone.

(2)   **Functions of the Frontal Lobe**

(a)   **Motor Cortex (Precentral Gyrus)**

Neurons in the motor cortex provide inten- tional, voluntary control of the skeletal muscles. A lesion of the motor cortex results in paralysis or paresis. The cortex has a function of inhibition as well as initiation of motor impulses. The precentral gyrus is called the primary motor strip. When an individual experiences damage to the motor cortex, he or she will experience varying degrees of inability to initiate movement, and the stretch reflex will not be inhibited (hyperreflexia).

i) **Homunculus (Projections)**

The motor cortex is arranged in a somatotopic pattern. Traditionally, anatomists draw an imaginary little person stretched out along the motor strip. This person is called the "homunculus." As seen from the distribution of the body of the "little man," there is almost an inverse relationship between the volume or area of the body part and its degree of cortical representation. The area of the motor cortex that supplies the legs, for example, is not significantly larger than the area that supplies the tongue. The implication is that there is a direct relationship between the amount of cortical representation of a structure and the extent of its nerve supply. In most cases, damage to a part of the homunculus in one hemisphere would result in paralysis, paresis, and/or paresthesia of that body part on the opposite (contralateral) side of the body. For example, a lesion in the area of cortical representation for the arm in the left cerebral hemisphere would result in paralysis, paresis and/or paresthesia of the right arm. Motor cortical representation to the head and neck is mostly bilateral, this means that both hemispheres provide voluntary motor control to both sides of the head and neck. Exceptions are the lower muscles of facial expression, the pharynx and the genioglossus muscles.

ii)   Decussation of Motor Tracts

Neurons from the motor cortex destined for the trunk and extremities decussate, or cross, at the trapezoid body in the lower medulla. Thus, neurons that originate (have their cell bodies) in the right hemisphere will have their effects on the opposite half of the body. The opposite side of the body is called contralateral. This holds for most of the muscles of the head, with certain exceptions. In the head and neck, some muscles receive contralateral innervation whereas others receive bilateral innervation.

(b)   Association Areas

i)   Premotor Cortex

The premotor cortex is responsible for organizing the plan for executing movements and transmits the plan to the primary motor cortex which is responsible for initiating voluntary contractions of the skeletal muscles. Damage to this area results in difficulty planning voluntary motor movements (apraxia).

ii)   Broca's Area (Pars Triangularis)

Programming of the complex voluntary movements associated with normal speech requires association with somesthetic, auditory, visual, and symbolic areas of the cortex. Broca's area is in the pars triangularis of the inferior frontal lobe. Damage to nerve cells here can result in apraxia. Apraxia also results from damage to somesthetic centers.

(c) **Other Functions**

Certain intellectual and personality functions appear to be related to the cortex of the frontal lobe. However, these functions are not entirely understood. Frontal lobotomy has been used to treat mental illness.

b. **Parietal Lobe**

The parietal lobe is generally associated with tactile reception and interpretation.

(1) **Location**

The parietal lobe lies beneath the parietal bone, posterior to the frontal lobe, superior to the temporal lobe and anterior to the occipital lobe.

(a) *Postcentral Gyrus:* The postcentral gyrus is posterior to the central fissure. It contains the somesthetic cortex.

(b) *Somesthetic Cortex (Sensory Cortex):* The somesthetic cortex, posterior to the central fissure, is associated with conscious tactile reception. There is a difference between conscious and unconscious sensory input; the postcentral strip receives conscious tactile sensations.

(2) **Functions**

(a) *Sensory Decussation:* Damage to the sensory cortex on one side results in paresthesia or anesthesia of the area on the opposite side.

(b) *Sensory Homunculus:* The sensory cortex is arranged somatotopically like the motor cortex.

(c) *Stereognosis:* The sensory cortex has association areas that interpret tactile input. The recognition and association of tactile input is stereognosis. Perception and discrimination of fine touch are essential to the learning of new spoken words.

(3)   Angular Gyrus

The angular gyrus is the seat of written language symbolization or representation. A lesion here might result in dyslexia.

(4)   Supramarginal Gyrus

The supramarginal gyrus is the seat of spoken language interpretation. Lesions here might result in Wernicke's aphasia (fluent aphasia), a condition in which the individual cannot symbolize properly and has difficulty understanding language. The patient with Wernicke's aphasia may also speak in jargon and have difficulty recalling words.

c.   **Temporal Lobe**

The temporal lobe is generally associated with auditory reception and interpretation. It has many intercortical connections, and not all of its functions are clear. It appears to be involved with integration of the cortex as a whole, in addition to its central auditory functions.

(1)   Location: The temporal lobe is located inferior to the lateral sulcus.

(a)   *Temporal Gyri:* There are three temporal lobe gyri: superior, middle, and inferior.

(b)   *Auditory Cortex (Heschl's Gyri):* The primary site for auditory reception is on the superior temporal gyrus. This area is known as Heschl's gyrus.

(2)   Functions

(a)   **Sensation (Reception)**

Speech-language pathologists and audiologists are interested in the various complexities of sensory processing. Auditory processing is a good example. Sensation is the most basic level of processing. It is nothing more than the awareness of the existence of a stimulus. To be sensed, the stimulus has to have sufficient intensity to trigger an action potential. Therefore, a patient with a lesion in the primary receptive areas of the temporal lobe might have difficulty becoming aware that an auditory stimulus was present, at all.

(b) **Perception**

Further up on the complexity chain is perception. Perception is complex but can be summarized in terms of distinguishing the characteristics of the stimulus. Acoustic characteristics include frequency, amplitude, and spectrum. These are perceived as pitch, loudness, and quality, respectively. Patients with lesions that affect auditory perception might have difficulty distinguishing one signal from another or distinguishing a signal from background noise.

(c) **Association**

Perhaps the highest level of sensory processing is association. At this level, some sort of meaning or relationship is attached to the input. Normal association requires input from memory. Patients with auditory association problems might have great difficulty pairing a spoken word with its linguistic referent.

(3) **Wernicke's Area**

Wernicke's area is the center for linguistic association of auditory, visual, and other signals. It is located at the junctures of the parietal, occipital, and temporal lobes. Lesions in Wernicke's area result in difficulty understanding spoken or written input, self-monitoring, and organization of output: aphasia.

d. **Occipital Lobe**

The occipital lobe is primarily associated with reception and association of visual impulses.

(1)   **Location:** It is located in the posterior portion of the brain.

    (a)   *Parieto-Occipital Fissure:* If you look at the medial surface of the hemisphere, the parieto-occipital sulcus (fissure) is clearly visible. This sulcus separates the parietal and occipital lobes.

    (b)   *Calcarine Fissure:* Here, we find the seat of the primary visual cortex, where visual stimuli are sensed. It is medial and inferior to the parieto-occipital sulcus.

    (c)   *Visual Cortex:* On either bank of the calcarine sulcus, we find the primary visual cortex. This is where visual impulses are received from the retinae and the optic nerve.

(2)   **Functions**

    (a)   **Sensation**

Visual functions are processed on the same levels as are auditory functions or any other special sensory function. Sensation is the awareness that a visual stimulus exists. Damage to the visual cortex causes differing degrees of cortical blindness.

        i)   *Retinal Projections:* The optic nerve fibers from the retinae project to discrete areas of the visual cortex. The visual field is upside down and backward.

        ii)   *Optic Decussation:* Decussation means crossing. About half of the fibers from the optic nerve cross at the optic chiasm, a prominent landmark on the inferior aspect of the brain, under the frontal lobe. The fibers that decussate originate at the rods and cones of the nasal side of the retina. Fibers that originate in the rods and cones of the inferior retina loop through the temporal lobe at Meyer's loop. Inferior fibers loop and nasal fibers cross.

iii) *Anopsia:* Because some fibers cross and some do not, a quadrantal arrangement of the visual pathways and cortex results. If there is disease or damage to discrete parts of these pathways or cortex, the result can be blindness in parts of the patient's visual field. These types of central visual deficits are called "anopsias," and can be called homonymous or heteronymous (on the same side or on opposite sides respectively), quadrantal (affecting 1/4 of the visual field), or hemianopsia, (affecting 1/2 of the visual field), depending on which portion of the visual field is affected.

(b) **Perception**

Recognition of a visual stimulus (perception) is accomplished by comparing it with other items in storage. Difficulty with visual perception is a type of visual agnosia.

(c) **Association**

Patients with visual association problems have difficulty pairing visually presented stimuli with other stored referential concepts.

4.   **Subcortical Structures**

a.   **Thalamus**

The thalamus is the relay center for all sensory input except smell. It also seems to play roles in affect. Lesions in the thalamus are associated with impaired reception and organization of sensory input and with affective disorders, such as personality disturbances.

(1)   *Location:* The thalamus is located deep to the cerebral cortex at the rostral end of the brainstem.

It is composed grossly of two halves. Each half lies on either side of the third ventricle.

(2)   *Structure:* The thalamus consists of a number of gray matter nuclei: anterior, medial, lateral, and ventral.

(3)   *Function:* The thalamus relays sensory information to the various special cortical areas. It also receives information from the cortex, and is the center for reception of primitive impulses of pain, temperature, and gross touch.

b.   **Hypothalamus**

The hypothalamus is located inferior to the thalamus. It forms the floor and parts of the lateral wall of the third ventricle. The hypothalamus is associated with regulation of certain visceral functions. Hypothalamic lesions result in an imbalance of metabolic processes. These lesions usually produce grave results.

c.   **Pineal Body**

The pineal body forms the dorsal wall of the third ventricle. It is also called the epiphysis.

d.   **Basal Nuclei (Striate Bodies)**

(1)   **Names:** Between the cortex and the thalamus are three groups of neurons called the basal nuclei. They include the caudate nucleus, putamen, and the globus pallidus. The names "basal ganglia," "basal nuclei," "striate bodies" and "corpora striata" are synonymous. Two other cell body groups, the substantia nigra and subthalamic nucleus, are associated with the basal nuclei.

(2)   **General Location:** The basal nuclei are located between the thalamus and the cerebral cortex. The substantia nigra and subthalamic nucleus are ventral to the thalamus.

(3)   **Structure:** The inner mass of gray matter fibers called the basal nuclei are located in the inferomedial region of the hemispheres. The basal nuclei are formed of gray (unmyelinated) fibers with special neurotransmitters. The basal nuclei are important

in the refinement of movement. They appear to accomplish their functions by regulation of gross impulses from other parts of the CNS. Perhaps this function is augmented by special synaptic properties.

(4) **Functions:** The basal nuclei function in a highly complex interactive manner with multisynaptic neuronal projections and circuits. They seem to enhance the smooth execution of movement and probably play a larger role in awareness and cognition. Lesions in the basal nuclei result in hypokinetic or hyperkinetic dysarthria or, in the case of cerebral palsy, athetosis.

5. **Brainstem**

a. **Location:** Caudal to the thalamus.

(1) *Midbrain*

(2) *Pons*

(3) *Medulla*

b. **Relationship to Spinal Cord:** The brainstem is the rostral extention of the spinal cord inside the skull.

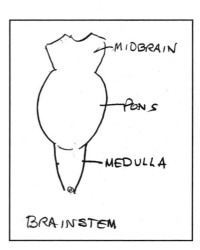

c. **Functions**

(1) **Ascending/Descending Tracts (CNS)**

(a) **Motor**
The lateral corticospinal tracts cross from one side to the other at the caudal medulla.

i) **Pyramidal:** Pyramidal tracts convey voluntary motor impulses from the motor cortex to the spinal and cranial nerves. They are the voluntary motor tracts that originate at the precentral gyrus. The corticospinal tracts, along with the corticobulbar tracts, are called the "pyramidal tracts," for two reasons. First, because the multipolar cell bodies in the precentral gyrus are shaped like irregular pyramids under microscopic examination. Second, because the places where the corticospinal tracts decussate, on either side of the medulla, are called pyramids by virtue of their macroscopic appearances. The crossing of the corticospinal tracts is known as the "decussation of the pyramids."

ii) **Extrapyramidal:** Extrapyramidal pathways relay and coordinate pyramidal functions with the subcortical structures and with the cerebellum. Extrapyramidal functions are passive and involuntary.

(b) **Sensory**

The sensory decussation is also in the medulla, just rostral to the motor decussation.

i) *Spinothalamic Tracts:* Spinothalamic tracts convey gross touch sensations, and cross at the segmental level.

ii) *Trigeminothalamic Tracts:* Trigeminothalamic tracts convey fine and gross touch from the face and anterior oral cavity. They are crossed and uncrossed.

iii) *Posterior Column Lemniscal Tracts:* The sensory tracts from the body convey touch sensations to the brain. Fine touch sensations are conveyed over the posterior column-lemniscal tracts. These tracts cross at the medulla level.

(c) *Decussations:* Two main crossings are located at the medulla level of the brainstem. These include the decussation of the pyramids and the sensory decussation. This means that discriminatory tactile impulses originating on the left side of the body are consciously received in the right cerebral hemisphere, and vice versa. Similarly, voluntary motor impulses originating in the left cerebral hemisphere are carried out on the right side of the body.

(d) **_Reticular System:_** The reticular system is a complex network of neurons that control the activation levels of the brain.

(e) **_Vestibular System:_** The vestibular system coordinates the muscular response of the body to impulses generated at the semicircular canals.

6. **Cerebellum**

a. **Location:** The cerebellum is connected to the brainstem at several levels. The cerebellum is located posterior-inferior to the cerebral hemispheres in the inferior cranial fossa.

b. **Function:** The functions of the cerebellum are passive. The cerebellum coordinates synergistic muscle functions through input from the muscles, brainstem, thalamus, and cerebral cortex.

7. **Meninges**

The entire CNS, including the brain, is enclosed in three layers of protective connective tissue called meninges.

a. **_Dura:_** The outermost layer is the dura mater (hard mother). It is a tough membrane designed to resist penetration. The space between the dura and the next layer is called the subdural space.

b. **_Arachnoid:_** The next layer is called the arachnoid mater (spider mother, "like a web"). It is a loose layer and forms a tenuous sleeve, for a short distance along nerves leaving the CNS. A fluid (cerebrospinal fluid) flows around the CNS in the space between the arachnoid mater and the next layer.

c.   *Pia:* The pia mater lies next to the brain. The name means nourishing mother. It is the matrix for blood vessels that spread out over the surface of the CNS. It also contains some fine fibers that appear to be associated with the autonomic nervous system.

8.   **Cerebrospinal Fluid (CSF)**

Cerebrospinal fluid (CSF) is the clear fluid that circulates in and around the entire central nervous system (CNS).

a.   **Composition:** It is composed of small quantities of inorganic salts and some proteins: potassium chloride, sodium chloride, albumin, and dextrose.

b.   **Function:** Cerebrospinal fluid plays several roles. It protects the CNS from shock, balances pressure changes brought about by changes in blood volume and postural changes, and functions like lymph.

c.   **Ventricles:** The first two ventricles are called the lateral ventricles. They are located deep in the cerebral hemi-spheres. The third ventricle is located between the halves of the thalamus, and the fourth ventricle is located in the brainstem.

d.   **Foramina:** Foramina (singular: foramen) are the holes through which the CSF flows. It flows from the lateral ventricles into the third ventricle through two interventric-ular foramina. CSF flows from the third ventricle through the cerebral aqueduct to the fourth ventricle. From the fourth ventricle, it flows into the subarachnoid space via two lateral and one medial foramina.

e.   **Subarachnoid Space:** From the fourth ventricle, the CSF escapes into the subarachnoiod space. This is the space between the arachnoid and pia mater.

f.   **Flow of Cerebrospinal Fluid:** Cerebrospinal fluid is formed in the ventricles. The greatest amount is produced by the choroid plexuses of the ventricles. The average volume of CSF in the adult is about 135 mL. The average volume secreted daily is about 550 mL. This means that the CSF is in total circulation and the total volume is replaced every six hours in the adult. CSF is absorbed by arachnoid villi in the area of the superior dural sagittal sinus. They transport the fluid into the superior sagittal sinus to return in the circulatory system with venous blood drainage.

B. **Spinal Cord in Detail**

1. **Structure**

The spinal cord is the extension of the CNS outside the skull. It consists of an outer layer of myelinated fiber bundles and an inner layer of unmyelinated neurons. The cord is contained in the vertebral canal of the spinal column. It is divided from the brain at the level of the foramen magnum. This is a geographic (rather than functional) landmark. This suggests that, anatomically, the spinal cord is just an extension of the brainstem (approximately 17 inches to L-1/L-2). The spinal cord is divided into sections that correspond roughly with vertebral sections; only spinal cord sections are called segments. There are 8 cervical segments, 12 thoracic segments, 5 lumbar, and 5 sacral segments, and 1 coccygeal segment. At the lower end, spinal segments and vertebral segments diverge. The infant cord nearly fills the entire length of the vertebral canal.

2. **Function**

The spinal cord is the main connection between the central nervous system and the trunk and extremities. Ascending and descending tracts convey conscious and unconscious action potentials to and from these structures. Injury to the spinal cord can result in disruption or cessation of functions in body parts served by segments caudal to the injury.

III. **Peripheral Nervous System**

A. **Spinal and Cranial Nerves**

Cranial nerves are distinct in that most of them have their cell bodies in the brainstem. Their axons run in a variety of directions, depending on their functions. Nerves that have their cell bodies (ganglia) aggregated near the foramen magnum have some rootlets emerging from the rostral portion of the spinal cord. The spinal nerves have their cell bodies on or near the spinal cord.

1.   12 Cranial Nerves

Cranial Nerve	Communicative Functions	S/M/B
I Olfactory	The role of smell in communication is not widely discussed. Perhaps it is best to think of smell as having an indirect effect on communication. Good smells can enhance communication and bad smells can inhibit it. The olfactory nerve has end organs that sense chemical changes in the environment, and action potentials generated by these organs are conveyed to the cerebral hemispheres to be interpreted as smell. The olfactory nerve has no output, and conveys its action potentials to the insular cortex	S
II Optic	End organs in the retinae of each eye generate action potentials that are conveyed to the thalamus. These impulses are either interpreted as vision, or are used to stimulate the involuntary reactions of the eyes. The communicative functions of vision are many. These include, reading and writing, and interpretation of gestures, sign language, and facial expressions	S
III Oculomotor	This nerve reacts to input from the optic nerve and from the voluntary eye field of the cerebral cortex to activate most of the extrinsic and all the intrinsic muscles of the eye. It also conveys input from the eye muscles back to the thalamus to coordinate the other eye movements. Its communicative functions include control of most of the orbital (extraocular) muscles for tracking. The oculomotor nerve also provides motor innervation for the levator palpebrae superiorus muscle. This is the muscle that lifts the upper eyelid and opens the eye. Disability in opening the eyes is called ptosis. The oculomotor nerve also controls the intrinsic muscles of the eye that effect control of accommodation (focusing the eye) and pupil dilation (light reflex). This nerve is given the "B" category because of its unconscious sensory function to coordinate contractions of IV and VI.	B
IV Trochlear	The trochlear nerve provides motor output and coordinated input for the superior oblique muscle. This extrinsic eye muscle causes the eye to look down and out. Thus, it assists in visual tracking for reading and for orienting to other environmental communicative signals. The trochlear nerve has an anatomic distinction that makes it easy to remember. It is the only cranial nerve to exit the dorsal aspect of the brainstem. It does this at the rostral pons level of the brainstem. It is also the only peripheral nerve that crosses. Thus, fiber crossing for IV occurs within the PNS. IV has sensory fibers to coordinate its function with III and VI.	B

Cranial Nerve	Communicative Functions	S/M/B
V Trigeminal	The trigeminal conveys motor impulses down and touch impulses up. It provides motor output to the muscles of mandibular elevation. These muscles have obvious roles in mastication. For speech purposes, elevation of the mandible is important in production of all the anterior consonants, all the closed vowels, and most of the front vowels. One need only depress the mandible to realize the limitations imposed on the range of possible phonemes. The trigeminal nerve also supplies motor innervation to the tensor veli palatini muscle, thus affecting nasal resonance. The trigeminal nerve conveys touch impulses from the surface of the face and from the interior of the mouth. Regions of touch on the superficial parts of the body are called dermatomes. Touch is very important because it allows the speaker to realize the position and movement status of the oral musculature and structures. This realization is conscious at first, but probably becomes unconscious in running speech. There are three facial areas of skin to convey touch sensations with the three branches of the trigeminal nerve. These are the ophthalmic, maxillary, and mandibular dermatomes. The maxillary dermatome also serves the upper interior of the oral cavity, and the mandibular dermatome applies to the inferior oral cavity, including the anterior 2/3 of the tongue	B
VI Abducens	The sixth cranial nerve supplies motor innervation to the lateral rectus muscle. This muscle pulls the eyeball to the side and out. Its communication importance lies in visual tracking. Note: Cranial Nerves III, IV, and VI operate in concert to provide motor innervation of the muscles of the eyes. These three nerves together are easy to remember and can be tested together by observing how a patient coordinates the movements of his or her eyes and how his or her pupils respond to accommodation or light changes. VI has sensory fibers to coordinate with III and IV.	B
VII Facial	The facial nerve has two functions. It conducts efferent motor action potentials from the CNS to the muscles of the facial expression. One sign of damage to the motor supply of these muscles is dropping of the lower muscles of facial expression. Motor impulses to the muscles of the facial expression are essential for: facial gestures, labial phonemes (formed through contraction of all or part of the orbicularis oris muscle. Rounded vowels also require contraction of the orbicularis oris muscle), and retention of oral fluids. Sometimes we can spot weakness of the orbicularis oris muscle by the presence of a light drool line at one or the other oral margins. This cranial nerve also conveys the sense of taste from the anterior 2/3 of the tongue. Taste may not be so important to communication, but it has a role in feeding and swallowing.	B

Cranial Nerve	Communicative Functions	S/M/B
VIII Vestibulo-cochlear	Audition is the sense of hearing. Speech and hearing are, of course, related. We need to hear ourselves speak in order to speak normally, and we need good listeners in order to have a purpose for speaking. Cranial nerve VIII also carries sensations associated with changes in the position of the head in space. This affects our sense of balance and our posture.	S
IX Glosso-pharyngeal	IX has connections and coordinates in function with the pharyngeal plexus of nerves, which includes the facial (VII) and vagus (X) nerves. Its greatest role is in conveying taste and touch sensations from the oropharynx to the CNS. It also has some motor function, probably in concert with the accessory branch of the XI. Thus, it assists with the pharyngeal stage of swallowing and also affects pharyngeal resonance. Another role of XI is to provide motor innervations to the parotid salivary gland. The integrity of this nerve is not easy to test; however, alteration in the perception of taste is common with glossopharyngeal nerve damage. With isolated glossopharyngeal nerve damage, the patient may complain of an inability to taste bitter substances.	B
X Vagus	The vagus nerve supplies smooth muscle motor function to the pharynx, thorax, and some abdominal muscles. Afferent functions of X include conscious and unconscious somesthesis in the pharynx and thorax.	B
XI Accessory	It is important to emphasize that voluntary contraction of the striated pharyngeal muscles, including the velopharynx and larynx, is a function of XI, not X. To that extent, X and XI, or even IX, X, and XI, should be regarded as a complex, because accurate muscle contraction depends, in part, on accurate somesthesis. Motor fibers of XI accompany X to supply voluntary innervations to the striated muscles of intrinsic muscles of the larynx, allowing a patient to phonate and protect the airway. Pharyngeal constrictors, altering vocal tract resonance and facilitating transfer of the food bolus to the esophagus. Palatal elevation, allowing coupling of the nasal cavity to the vocal tract. Remember, though, that the trigeminal nerve supplies motor innervations to the tensor veli palatine muscle. We can screen Xth nerve function by listening to our patients' voices. If they sound breathy, the implication is of incomplete vocal fold adduction. This could be cause by vocal fold paralysis or paresis due to damage to CN X. Damage to the vagus nerve may also lead to aspiration risk as full adduction of the vocal folds helps protect the airway during swallowing. The XIth nerve provides motor innervations to the sternocleidomastoid and the upper portion of the trapezius. When this nerve is damaged, the individual may have difficulty independently supporting his or her head. Head position is important in swallowing and adaptive equipment may be necessary to help reduce the risk of aspiration if the patient presents with swallowing difficulties and has cranial nerve XI damage.	M

Cranial Nerve	Communicative Functions	S/M/B
XII Hypoglossal	This nerve is the final common pathway for motor innervations to the intrinsic and most of the extrinsic tongue muscles. The exception is the palatoglossus muscle, which receives innervations from the pharyngeal plexus. We can easily appreciate how movements of the tongue are important to speaking and swallowing.	M

(1)   **31 Spinal Nerves**

Thirty-one pairs of spinal nerves have their cell bodies in the ventral horns of the spinal cord or in the dorsal root ganglia, near the cord. These nerves correspond to spinal cord segments, and to 31 embryonic somatic segments. The 31 spinal nerves have roles in communication. Their most important one for speech is to allow expansion of the thoracic cavity in respiration. The primary muscle of inspiration is the diaphragm, innervated by the phrenic nerves, one on each side. These nerves receive fibers from the cervical plexus, arising from C3, C4, and C5 spinal cord segments. The external intercostals and accessory inspiratory and expiratory muscles are innervated at the thoracic spinal segments Gestures and writing are also important forms of communication, and motor innervation of the upper extremities is provided through the nerves of the brachial plexus. These nerves arise from spinal segments C5, C6, C7, C8, and T1. The extent to which the lower extremities play communicative roles is probably applied through the role of ambulation in language development. Nerves of the lumbar and sacral plexuses are associated with lower extremity function.

B.   **Autonomic Nervous System (Ganglia and Nerve Processes)**

The autonomic nervous system (ANS) is primarily an efferent system that supplies smooth muscle, cardiac muscle, and glands. It responds to diffuse internal and external stimuli. Central nervous system connections to the ANS are provided by preganglionic connector neurons, with cell bodies in the brainstem and spinal cord. These connect to postganglionic effector neurons, which supply the various visceral, cardiac, and glandular organs. Postganglionic effector neurons have cell bodies in diverse autonomic ganglia.

1. **Sympathetic**

    a. *Thoracolumbar Outflow:* Sympathetic preganglionic connector neurons cell bodies are in thoracic and lumbar spinal cord segments.

    b. *Emergency Actions:* The sympathetic division activates emergency unconscious bodily reactions, like secretion of adrenalin or opening of the arterial lumen.

2. **Parasympathetic**

    a. *Craniosacral Outflow:* Parasympathetic preganglionic connector neurons have cell bodies in the brainstem and sacral spinal cord segments.

    b. *Normal Bodily Functions:* The parasympathetic division regulates normal unconscious bodily functions such as digestion.

UNIT 7

THE AUDITORY SYSTEM

I.   **Two Main Divisions of the Human Auditory System**

    A.   **Peripheral Auditory System**

        1.   *Location and Extent:* The peripheral system includes all the structures from the outer ear, or pinna, to and including the acoustic nerve.

        2.   *Functions:* The peripheral nervous system has three functions: It selectively amplifies acoustic energy from the environment, aids in localization of a sound source, and transforms acoustic energy into neurochemical potentials.

    B.   **Central Auditory System**

        1.   *Location and Extent:* The central auditory system includes the neural pathways through which sound sensation impulses are transmitted from the level of the brainstem to the cerebral cortex.

        2.   *Functions:* The central auditory system processes impulses from the peripheral system for perception.

II.   **The Peripheral Hearing Mechanism in Detail**

    A.   **External (Outer) Ear**

        1.   **Pinna (Auricle)**

            a.   *Form*

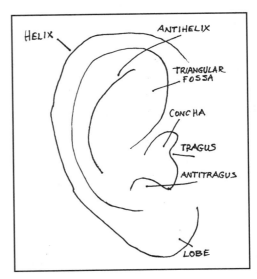

                (1)   Helix

                (2)   Antihelix

                (3)   Tragus

                (4)   Antitragus

                (5)   Lobe

                (6)   Concha

                (7)   Triangular Fossa

            b.   *Functions of the Pinna:* The pinna acts as a collector for acoustic energy and may play a role in the localization of sound. We appear to be slightly more sensitive to sound delivered to the front of our heads than we are to sound delivered to the back. The localization function may be accomplished though a shadow effect, with acoustic energy casting a shadow behind the pinna.

2. **External Auditory Meatus (EAM)**

The external auditory meatus is also called the ear canal. It is the conduit whereby acoustic energy is propagated to the sensitive receptors of the inner ear.

a. **Form:** The external auditory meatus is "S"-shaped, and extends from the pinna to the tympanic membrane. Its acoustic function is to collect and selectively amplify sound. The biological function of the external auditory meatus is protective.

    (1) **Ear Canal**

        (a) *Shape:* Its bony portion (proximal 2/3) protects the delicate structures of the middle ear from damage by trauma or dirt, and so forth.

        (b) *Underlying Tissue Composition:* The distal one-third of the external auditory meatus (EAM) is skin-covered cartilage, and the proximal two-thirds is skin-covered bone.

        (c) *Cerumen:* The cartilaginous distal one-third enables one to insert objects into the canal, such as hearing aid ear molds, or ear plugs. The skin over the cartilaginous portion contains a protective mechanism. This mechanism is composed of hair follicles, sebaceous (oil-secreting), and ceruminous (ear wax-secreting) glands. Cerumen is a waxy substance which helps maintain the acidic environment of the external auditory meatus and entraps physical objects.

    (2) **Tympanic Membrane**

    The tympanic membrane (TM) could be considered part of either the outer or the middle ear. The inner lamina tissue is continuous with the tissue of the tympanum, and the tissue of the outer lamina is continuous with that of the EAM. In form, the TM is a conical, translucent membrane about 9 mm in diameter.

(a)   ***Laminae:*** It is made up of four layers of tissue. The outer and inner layers are continuous with the tissues of the EAM and the tympanum, respectively. The middle layers are grained with concentric circles (inner), and with radial striations (outer). They provide support and enhance sound transmission.

(b)   ***Pars Tensa:*** The largest part of the tympanic membrane is tightly suspended and plays the major role in the transmission of acoustic energy to the middle ear.

(c)   ***Pars Flaccida:*** In the upper anterior area of each tympanic membrane is a little cul de sac called the notch of Rivinius. Here, the fibers are sparser, and the membrane is not as tightly rigged. This area appears to have a role in pressure equalization for the tympanic cavity.

d)   ***Otoscopic Landmarks***
   - Pars Tensa
   - Pars Flaccida
   - Malleolar Stria

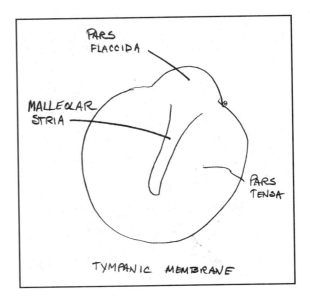

b. **Functions**

(3) *Acoustic Function:* The external ear collects and selectively amplifies sound. It is a tube with one open end; it will amplify sounds according to its length.

(4) *Protective Function:* The bony portion (proximal two-thirds) protects the delicate structures of the middle ear from damage by trauma or dirt, and so on. The cartilaginous distal one-third enables one to insert objects into the canal, such as hearing aid ear molds or earplugs. As noted above, the skin over the cartilaginous portion contains a protective mechanism. This mechanism is composed of hair follicles, sebaceous (oil-secreting), and ceruminous (ear wax-secreting) glands. Cerumen is a waxy substance that helps maintain the acidic environment of the external auditory meatus as well as entraps physical objects.

c. **Mastoid Process (of Temporal Bone)**

The mastoid process of the temporal bone is posterior/inferior to the pinna. The air cells of the temporal bone are porous. This bone is a site for application of bone vibrators for auditory stimulus delivery. This is a way to examine the sensitivity of the cochlea without involving the external and middle ears.

B. **Middle Ear (Tympanum)**

1. *General Form and Extent:* The middle ear is an air-filled cavity extending from the tympanic membrane to the bony capsule of the inner ear. Its volume is 1 to 2 cm^3. Its main dimensions are the tympanic cavity, the epitympanic recess (where the head of the malleus is situated), and the additus which maintains open communication with mastoid air cells. The term "eardrum" is properly applied to the entire middle ear, not just the membrane. The drumhead is the membrane. It also seals the middle ear from the air in the EAM.

2. *Function:* The middle ear separates the external ear from the delicate structures of the inner ear. It also amplifies the acoustic energy delivered to the tympanic membrane.

3.   **Structures of the Middle Ear**

   a.   **Tympanic Membrane**

   The TM is a conical, translucent membrane about 9 mm in diameter.

   (1)   *Structure:* It is made up of four layers of tissue. The outer and inner layers are continuous with the tissues of the EAM and the tympanum, respectively. The middle layers are grained with concentric circles (inner) and with radial striations (outer). The middle layers provide support and enhance sound transmission.

   (2)   *Function:* Most of the TM is tight, with many fibers. It vibrates in unison with the sound source. The pars flaccida of the TM assists in pressure equalization.

   b.   **Ossicles**

   These are the tiny bones of the middle ear that form the ossicular chain. They are the smallest bones in the body.

   (1)   **Form**

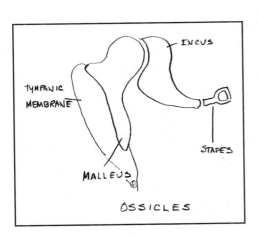

   (a)   *Malleus:* The malleus is the most distal or lateral of the ossicular bones. It is shaped like a hammer with a long portion called the manubrium or handle, and a rounded head. The malleus is attached to the tympanic membrane from its conical tip (umbo) to its posterosuperior margin.

   (b)   *Incus:* The incus is the middle bone in the ossicular chain. It articulates with the malleus. There is very little movement between them. Incus means "anvil."

   (c)   *Stapes:* The stapes articulates with the incus at the smallest synovial joint in the body (incudostapedial). Stapes means "stirrup." Its footplate fits into the oval window of the cochlea.

(2) **Impedance Matching Function**

The area of the tympanic membrane is about 17 times greater than that of the oval window. Thus, the ossicles act like a wedge to concentrate the force of the sound pressure at the TM into a greater pressure at the oval window. There is a lever action inherent in the action of the bones' articulation (Goode et al., 1994).

c. **Eustachian (Pharyngotympanic) Tubes**

(1) *Structure and Location:* Tubes run from the anterior parts of each tympanum to the posterior-lateral nasopharyngeal wall at the superior conchae level. They are composed of mucous membrane tissue surrounded by elastic cartilage (inner 2/3) and bone (1/3 nearest the tympanum).

(2) *Function:* The eustachian tubes function to provide pressure equalization for the middle ears. They are normally closed except during swallowing when they open for a brief time. They also open when there is a large pressure differential between the middle ears and the outside environment. The salpingopharyngeus muscles elevate the pharynx and open the eustachian tubes during swallowing. Under pathologic conditions, the eustachian tubes become swollen and lose their patency (patent = open). The result may be middle ear pathology.

d. **Muscles of the Middle Ear**

The ossicles are supported with a system of muscles and tendons. This suspension plays a role in how they function.

(1) *Stapedius:* The stapedius muscle arises (originates) in a bony canal in the posterior area of the tympanic cavity and inserts via a long tendon at the head of the stapedius.

(2) *Tensor Tympani:* The tensor tympani originates in a canal in the anterior tympanic wall, parallel with the eustachian tube, and inserts into the manubrium of the malleus. It is the larger of the tympanic muscles (about 25 mm in length).

(3)   *Acoustic Reflex:* The acoustic reflex occurs when the muscles contract in response to loud sounds. This reflex appears to attenuate acoustic energy delivered to the oval window. The acoustic reflex has a role in audiologic testing. Much discussion has concerned the role of the acoustic reflex in protecting the inner ear from damage produced by high amplitude environmental acoustic sources. Zemlin (1998) reviewed the literature and concluded that the acoustic reflex provided little, if any, such protection.

4.   **Middle Ear Function Testing**

- Middle ear function is important for proper conduction of sound to the inner ear. Equal pressure on both sides of the tympanic membrane is necessary for optimum tympanic function. Otologists, audiologists, and others examine the external and middle portions of the ear visually with an instrument called an otoscope. The otoscope allows visual inspection of the tympanic membrane, the first step in tympanic assessment. Otoscopic examination can reveal the patency of the ear canal, the structural integrity of the tympanic membrane, and the presence of fluid medial to that membrane. Special attachments to the otoscope can also provide a preliminary look at tympanic mobility by varying the air pressure in the ear canal.

- Audiologists derive a preliminary assessment of tympanic function by comparing air conduction pure tone thresholds with bone conduction thresholds. Normally, both are equivalent. If there is a conductive hearing loss, bone conduction thresholds are usually lower. In the absence of external auditory meatus obstruction, the primary suspect for conductive loss would be the tympanum.

- Acoustic impedance testing is the most important means of assessing tympanic function. Audiologists use tympanometry to verify the tympanic efficiency in transferring sound to the inner ear.

C.   **Inner Ear (Labyrinth)**

1.   *Location:* It is located in the petrous portion of the temporal bone.

2.   *Bony Labyrinth:* The bony labyrinth is located within the bony portion of the temporal bone. It is named after a mythical (Greek)

trap into which the hero, Icarus, was imprisoned. The bony labyrinth of the temporal bone is a series of tunnels of different sizes hollowed out of the bone. There are two series of tunnels: one for hearing (cochlea) and one for balance (semicircular canals). They are connected to the vestibule, a central structure. The vestibule contains the receptor cells for the sense of balance.

3. *Membranous Labyrinth:* The soft tissue within the bony labyrinth is called the membranous labyrinth.

4. **Inner Ear Structures**

    a. **Hearing Mechanism**

        The structure that serves the sense of hearing in the labyrinth is the cochlea.

        (1) **Cochlea:** The cochlea has no external structure except that of the bone in which it is located.

            (a) *Shape:* Resembling a snail's shell, it is a spiral with 2¾ turns (in human beings). Unwound, it would be about 35 mm in length.

                i) *Basal End:* The end nearest the ossicles is the basal end. The scala vestibuli connects to the vestibule at its basal end. The scala tympani connects to the tympanum (round window) at its basal end.

                ii) *Apical End:* The end at the tip is the apical end. The scalae connect there at the helicotrema.

            (b) *Membranous Portion of the Cochlea:* The cochlear membranes are divided into three stairways (so called because they wind around like a spiral staircase).

                i) **Scala Media**

                    a) *Endolymph:* The scala media is filled with and surrounded by fluids. The fluid inside the cochlear duct is endolymph.

It protects the delicate inner structures and aids in acoustic energy transmission.

b) *Perilymph:* The fluid outside the scala media is perilymph. It protects the scala media from the bony labyrinth and aids in acoustic energy transmission.

ii) **Basilar Membrane:** The basilar membrane is the structure in the scala media on which the sensory structures are located. It also separates the scala media from the scala tympani.

a) *Organ of Corti:* The organ of Corti is located on the basilar membrane. It contains the sensory receptor cells for hearing called hair cells.

b) *Stereocilia (Hair Cells):* These are the cells that convert acoustic energy into neuro-chemical potentials. There are four rows: The inner row contains about 3,500 cells, and three outer rows contain about 20,000 cells. The hair cells touch the tectorial membrane all along the spiral of the scala media. We do not fully understand how the hair cells convert acoustic energy into neural potential. The functions of the hair cells in the basilar membrane are to respond differentially to acoustic energy bandwidths in the audible spectrum and to convert that energy into neural impulses.

c) *Tectorial Membrane:* The tectorial membrane hangs over the organ of Corti along its entire length. The hair cells touch this membrane.

d) *Spiral Ganglion:* The hair cells are connected to one another by nerve fibers. These fibers combine to form the spiral ganglion. The auditory nerve is formed by the fibers of the spiral ganglion. This is the hearing branch of the vestibulocochlear nerve (VIII).

iii) **Reissner's (Vestibular) Membrane:** Reissner's membrane separates the scala media from the scala vestibuli.

(c) *Bony Portion of the Cochlea*

i) *Scala Tympani:* Lies inferior to the scala media. It is filled with periymph.

ii) *Scala Vestibuli:* Superior to scala media. It is filled with perilymph.

iii) *Helicotrema:* The hole that allows the scala tympani to connect to the scala vestibuli.

iv) *Modiolus:* The bony inner structure of the cochlea.

(2) **Cochlear Nerve**

(a) *Cranial Nerve VIII: Auditory Division:* This division conveys neural impulses to the thalamus and on into the cerebral cortex where they will be interpreted as sound.

i) *Cochlear Nerve Nuclei:* Here the VIIIth nerve synapses with the brainstem. At this point, we leave the peripheral auditory system. There is a ventral cochlear nucleus and a dorsal cochlear nucleus.

ii)   *Cochlear Nuclear Synapses:* The VIIIth nerve fibers bifurcate and synapse with the cochlear nuclei. One branch synapses at the dorsal cochlear nucleus and the other branch is destined for the ventral cochlear nucleus. The branch headed for the ventral cochlear nucleus bifurcates again, sending potentials to the anteroventral and posteroventral divisions of the ventral cochlear nucleus.

b.   **Vestibular Mechanism (System)**

- The vestibular mechanism interprets changes in position of the body to convey the sense of balance. It is composed of the noncochlear parts of the bony labyrinth in the petrous portion of the temporal bone. These parts are called the semicircular canals, the utricle, and the saccule.

- The vestibular apparatus has sensory receptors in the semicircular canals, the utricle, and the saccule, all of which communicate with the cochlea. There is great interconnectivity between the vestibular apparatus, brainstem nuclei, spinal cord, and the cerebellum.

(1)   *Utricle:* A bony, membrane-lined pouch connected to the semicircular canals. It appears to sense acceleration in the horizontal or axial plane.

(2)   *Saccule:* Smaller than the utricle, the saccule communicates with the scala vestibuli of the cochlea, and appears to sense acceleration in the vertical plane.

(3)   *Central Structure of Labyrinth:* The point at which inner ear structures connect.

(4)   *Semicircular Canals:* There are three semicircular canals in the petrous portion of the temporal bone. These contain sensory membranes, which respond to the head's position in space.

(a) Vertical Canals

    i) Anterior vertical canals

    ii) Posterior vertical canals

(b) Horizontal Canal

c. **Inner Ear Functions**

(1) **Functions for Hearing Mechanism**

(a) *Basilar Membrane:* The basilar membrane contains sensory end organs that respond to acoustic energy.

    i) *Frequency Analysis:* At its apical end, the basilar membrane's sensory organs are more sensitive to lower energy frequencies. Near the basilar end, where the stapes footplate enters the oval window, the membrane is most sensitive to higher frequencies.

    ii) *Transduction:* End organs in the basilar membrane are called stereocilia ("hair cells"). These are ciliated neuroepithelial cells that generate action potentials in response to cochlear fluid vibrations. Action potentials generated by hair cells are propagated to the auditory nerve.

(b) *Auditory Nerve:* The auditory nerve is the cochlear division of cranial nerve VIII. Cell bodies of its bipolar neurons are located in the spiral ganglion, which follows the 2¾ spiral winds of the basilar membrane.

    i) *Threshold:* Auditory threshold is the minimum stimulus intensity that elicits a response from the patient to one-half the presentations.

    ii) *Firing Rate of the Nerve:* Loudness, a perceptual phenomenon associated with sound pressure levels, appears to be generally associated with auditory nerve firing rate. Increases in sound amplitude evoke higher numbers of auditory neuron action potential spikes per unit time. There remains some controversy regarding this matter.

iii)   *Frequency Perception:* Pitch, a perceptual phenomenon, is the psychologic correlate of acoustic energy frequency. Because locations on the basilar membrane are differentially sensitive to frequency, specific (inner) hair cells stimulated by a given frequency begin the complex process of pitch discrimination.

iv)   *Temporal Perception:* Temporal perception is the psychologic correlate of stimulus duration and interstimulus interval. It is a topic of much interest to language researchers.

(2)   **Functions of Vestibular Mechanism**

(a)   *Perception of Position in Space:* Sensory organs of the vestibular mechanism respond to changes in head position and to acceleration.

(b)   *Relationship to Extraocular Muscles:* The vestibular mechanism is closely related to the extrinsic eye muscles. Their coordination preserves stability of visual perception as the individual moves about.

(c)   *Relationship to Muscles of Posture and Locomotion:* A functional relationship between the vestibular system and the postural muscles enables the individual to maintain a positional attitude during movement.

II. **The Central Auditory System**

A. **Location and Limits**

The central auditory system includes the neural pathways through which sound sensation impulses are transmitted from the level of the brainstem to the cerebral cortex. Its function is to process auditory impulses from the peripheral system for perception. Not all central auditory functions are conscious. There are unconscious centers in the central auditory system, which trigger certain unconscious reflexes such as hearing orientation and the muscular reflexes of the middle ear.

B. **Structures of the Central Auditory System**

1. *Brainstem Structures*

The central auditory system begins at the caudal pons in the ventral and dorsal cochlear nuclei. It should be emphasized that cranial nerve VIII is part of the peripheral auditory system.

a. *Pons:* Cochlear nuclei have synapses located roughly where the cerebellum and the pons connect. The rostral end of the trapezoid body is located in the pons, as well. Here, most auditory fibers decussate.

b. *Midbrain:* The midbrain has an important center for audition. It is called the inferior colliculus. There is an inferior colliculus in the right and one on the left. In the midbrain, some auditory fibers connect to centers for unconscious processing, such as those that trigger the stapedial reflex.

2. *Thalamus*

All sensory inputs except smell have relay centers in the thalamus. The thalamic center for hearing is the medial geniculate nucleus.

3. **Cerebral Cortex**

The primary receptive site for auditory stimuli is in the temporal lobe.

a. *Heschl's Gyrus:* Heschl's gyrus is the primary temporal lobe receptive site for auditory stimuli. One is located in the middle of the superior temporal gyrus of each hemisphere.

b. *Association Areas:* Cortical association areas for auditory processing are those areas that involve increasingly more complex processing. From frequency and quality differentiation to symbolic representation and storage, association areas coordinate the functions of diverse cerebral centers. Studies of living subjects reported activity of the superior gyri of the temporal lobes upon presentation of sound stimuli. (Penfield & Roberts, 1959, pp. 2281–2287).

C. **Functions of the Central Auditory System: The Central Auditory Pathways**

- The auditory evoked response is now a standard means of examining central auditory system function.

- Surface electrodes are placed on the scalp, usually at the vertex of the skull. A stimulus, usually a "click" or some other transient aperiodic sound, is presented through headphones to an ear or to both ears.

- The stimulus is presented many times, and the results are summed. The sums are automatically recorded on a strip of paper. This recording paper is calibrated to display the measurement of time elapsed between stimulus presentation and the electrical activity associated with synaptic junction excitation. Examiners *infer* recorded peaks of electrical activity are created when the action potential crosses synaptic clefts at the sites along the auditory pathways: cochlear nuclei, superior olivary complex, lateral lemniscal nucleus, inferior colliculus, and medial geniculate body.

- It can take up to 300 msec for a stimulus-generated action potential, called the *auditory evoked response* or *AER*, to reach the brain. Naturally, it takes less time for the potentials to reach more caudal structures. AERs recorded at the lower levels of the central system are called BSERs (*brainstem evoked responses*).

1. **Brainstem**

   a. **Pons**

      (1) *Cochlear Nuclei*

      The central auditory system begins at the connections of the vestibulocochlear nerve (VIII) with the brainstem. These connections are at the cochlear nuclei. Cochlear nuclei have synapses located roughly where the cerebellum and the pons connect. This area is called the cerebellopontine junction. The auditory nerve divides into two sections (bifurcates) at this junction. One branch goes to the dorsal cochlear nucleus and the other to the ventral cochlear nucleus.

(a) *Dorsal Cochlear Nucleus:* The dorsal cochlear nucleus is the target of one branch of the auditory nerve.

(b) *Ventral Cochlear Nucleus:* The other branch of the auditory nerve synapses in the ventral cochlear nucleus. It further branches to the anteroventral cochlear nucleus and the posteroventral cochlear nucleus.

(c) *Tonotopic Representation:* The arrangement of neurons in a frequency-specific pattern. Tonotopic arrangement of neurons begins at the hair cells in the basilar membrane and appears to persist to the cerebral cortex. Tonotopic regions of the basilar membrane represent frequencies of sound energy in the audible range from about 20 Hz to about 20,000 Hz for humans.

(2) **Superior Olivary Complex**

The suerior olivary complex receives fibers from the cochlear nuclei (the anterior part of the ventral cochlear nucleus) for the transmission of sound sensations. It is located at the rostral end of a region where many nerve fiber tracts cross from one side of the body to the other side.

(a) *Decussation:* Between the cochlear nuclei and the superior olivary complex, about 85% of the nerve fibers cross from one side to the other side (decussate); the rest ascend ipsilaterally. That is, most sound impulses transmitted to the left ear will be sent to the right cerebral cortex. This decussation occurs at the trapezoid body. The trapezoid body is a large complex of axons and some nuclei that begins in the lower medulla and reaches rostrally to the caudal pons.

(b)   ***Localization of Sound Source:*** Localization of sound is facilitated by the auditory sense, phase, and other temporal onset differences. This localization and tracking of acoustic sources is sorted out by the decussation of nerve fibers in the trapezoid.

(c)   ***Olivocochlear Tracts:*** Some nerve fibers originate in the brainstem and propogate to the cochlea. These efferent potentials are fired through fibers that originate at the superior olive. This tract of fibers is called the olivocochlear fiber bundle tract.

b.   **Midbrain**

(1)   **Lateral Lemniscus**

The tract that carries sound generated action potentials to the inferious colliculus in the midbrain and on up to the medial geniculate nucleus in the thalamus. A lemniscus is a bundle of axons. The lateral lemniscus originates just above the superior olivary complex.

(a)   ***Inferior Colliculus:*** The axons of the lateral lemniscus converge at the inferior colliculus on the dorsal aspect of the midbrain. The inferior colliculus projects fibers to the medial geniculate body in the thalamus and thus is a central way station in the central auditory system. It is also heavily connected to other brainstem nuclei and is the relay center for reflexive responses to sound.

(b)   ***Nucleus of the Lateral Lemniscus:*** The nucleus of the lateral lemniscus is a collection of neuronal cell bodies in the upper portion of the lateral lemniscus. As a general term, a nucleus is a collection of neuronal cell bodies in the central nervous system (CNS). Some, but not all, lateral lemniscal fibers synapse at the lateral lemniscal nucleus.

(c)   ***Olivocochlear Bundle Fibers:*** Audiologists can estimate cochlear function through measurement of otoacoustic emissions. Otoacoustic emissions are sounds produced by vibrating hair cells. These emissions can be detected by modern sensitive microphones. Olivocochlear tracts are efferent tracts of the auditory system. Their function is not clear, but some theories posit that they play one or more roles in signal enhancement.

(2) **Association with Other Functions**

There are interconnections with the visual tracts and with the motor system in the midbrain. These interconnections are believed to provide the basis for orienting responses.

2. **Thalamus**

a. *Location:* The two halves of the thalamus are located deep in the cerebral hemispheres. They surround the third ventricle.

b. *General Function*

(1) *Sensory:* The general function of the thalamus is to serve as a relay and integration center for sensory input. All sensory input except olfaction have centers in the thalamus.

(2) *Emotional:* The thalamus and hypothalamus are heavily connected to the prefrontal cortex. Together they are believed to have some role in the integration of somatic and visceral functions, and in affective behavior.

c. *Medial Geniculate Body:* The thalamic relay center for audition is the medial geniculate body (nucleus). A nucleus is an aggregation of neuronal cell bodies in the central nervous system.

3. **Cerebral Cortex**

Meaningful auditory stimuli are processed in the linguistic centers of the cortex. These centers are much more diverse than those which process nonmeaningful input.

a. ***Temporal Lobe:*** The temporal lobes of the cerebral hemispheres are the destinations for action potentials to be interpreted as sound.

    (1) ***Heschl's Gyrus:*** Heschl's gyrus is the primary cerebral cortical receptive site for auditory action potentials. Here, the brain is aware that a sound exists, but does little to distinguish or interpret the sound. There is one on each hemisphere. It is located approximately in the center of the superior temporal gyrus and extends slightly onto the lateral and opercular surfaces.

    (2) ***Association Areas:*** Perception of auditory impulses is processed at cerebral cortical areas located away from Heschl's gyrus. The auditory association area is located in the posterior two-thirds of the superior temporal gyrus and the planum temporale.

    (3) ***Interaction with Other Cortical Functions:*** At the higher levels of processing, association fibers in the cerebral cortex bring other cerebral functions into play. Other senses, for example, as well as memory centers, are believed to be tapped for perceptual purposes.

b. ***Interhemispheric Differences:*** In most people, one cerebral hemisphere is "dominant" and the other is "non-dominant." There are differences in the way these two hemispheres process auditory stimuli.

    (1) ***Sensation:*** Sensation is the mere awareness that an auditory stimulus has occurred. The minimum amplitude required for a person to indicate sensation of a sound half the time is called the "threshold" for that sound.

    (2) ***Perception:*** Perception is what the brain does with a raw signal after it receives it. There are several more complex levels of perception, ranging from the discrimination of larger and smaller differences in signals to selective attention to single character-istics of a complex signal, and beyond, including linguistic processing.

(a) *Perception of Speech:* There appears to be a preference for segmental features of speech in the dominant cerebral hemisphere and for the suprasegmental aspects of speech in the nondominant hemisphere.

(b) *Perception of Other Stimuli:* The nondominant hemisphere appears to have a preference for processing musical stimuli.

(3) *Auditory Discrimination:* Discrimination is the appreciation of fine differences between similar stimuli. Auditory discrimination, then, is the awareness of differences between similar sounds.

(a) *Of General Acoustic Stimuli:* Auditory discrimination includes the ability to distinguish the differences between a bell and a whistle.

(b) *Of Speech Stimuli:* Speech discrimination is a special kind of auditory discrimination. It includes the ability to distinguish words such as "boat" and "coat."

c. *Auditory Memory:* Auditory memory is the storage and retrieval of information for future use.

REFERENCES AND RECOMMENDED READINGS

Anderson, K. (Ed.). (1994). *Mosby's medical, nursing, and allied health dictionary.* St. Louis, MO: Mosby-Year Book.

Brookes, M., & Zietman, A. (1998). *Clinical embryology: A color atlas and text.* Washington, DC: CRC Press.

Charpied, G. L. (2007). The par interna/media anatomy and histology in the human larynx. *Folia Phoniatrica, 59,* 241–249.

Clemente, C. (1975). *Anatomy: A regional atlas of the human body.* Philadelphia, PA: Lea & Febiger.

Culbertson, W. R., & Tanner, D. C. (2011). *The anatomy and physiology of speech and swallowing.* Dubuque, IA: Kendall Hunt.

Daniloff, R., Schuckers, G., & Feth, L. (1980). *The physiology of speech and hearing.* Englewood, Cliffs, NJ: Prentice-Hall.

Goode, R. L., Killion, M., Nakamura, K., & Nishihara, S. (1994). New knowledge about the function of the human middle ear: Development of an improved analog model. *American Journal of Otology, 15,* 145–154.

Hafen, B., & Karren, K. (1989). *Prehospital emergency care and crisis intervention.* Englewood, CO: Morton.

Hamilton, W. (1977). *Textbook of human anatomy.* Saint Louis, MO: C.V. Mosby.

Katz, J. (1994). *Handbook of clinical audiology.* Baltimore, MD: Williams and Wilkins.

Larsen, W. J. (2001). *Human embryology* (3rd ed.). New York, NY: Churchill Livingstone.

Martin, F. (1994). *Introduction to audiology* (5th ed.). Englewood Cliffs, NJ: Prentice-Hall.

Minifie, F., Hixon, T., & Williams, F. (1973). *Normal aspects of speech, hearing, and language.* Englewood Cliffs, NJ: Prentice-Hall.

Penfield, W., & Roberts, L. (1959). *Speech and brain mechanisms.* Princeton, NJ: Princeton University Press.

Ojemann, G. (1991). Cortical organization of language. *Journal of Neuroscience, 11,* 2281–2287.

Romanes, G. (Ed.). (1972). *Cunningham's textbook of anatomy* (11th ed.). London, UK: Oxford University Press.

Saito, H., & Itoh, I. (2003). Three-dimensional architecture of the intrinsic tongue muscles, particularly the longitudinal muscle, by the chemical-maceration method. *Anatomical Science International, 78*(3), 168–176.

Thomas, C. (Ed.). (1973). *Taber's cyclopedic medical dictionary.* Philadelphia, PA: F. A. Davis Company.

Van Riper, C., & Erickson, R. (1996). *Speech correction: An introduction to speech pathology and audiology* (9th ed.). Needham Heights, MA: Allyn & Bacon.

Zemlin, W. (1994). *Speech and hearing science: Anatomy and physiology* (4th ed.). Englewood Cliffs, NJ: Prentice-Hall.

Zemlin, W. R. (1998). *Speech and hearing science anatomy and physiology* (4th ed.). Needham Heights, MA: Allyn & Bacon.

ANSWERS TO SELF-TESTS

1.   Erect, facing the observer; front; directed toward the observer; at the sides

2.   Physiology

3.   Coronal

4.   Transverse

5.   Superior

6.   Inferior or distal

7.   Distal

8.   Lateral

9.   Inferior or distal

10.   Anatomy

11.   Geriatric

12.   Developmental

13.   Pathologic

14.   Experimental

1. Protoplasm

2. Growth; reproduction; metabolism; adaptation

3. Histology

4. Nucleus

5. a) Nervous; b) Epithelial; c) Muscle; d) Connective; e) Nervous

6. a) Ectoderm; b) Mesoderm; c) Ectoderm; d) Mesoderm; e) Endoderm (Entoderm).

7. Mandible and hyoid bones; thyroid and cricoid cartilages.

8. Intake of food water and air.

9. Germ layers

10. Diarthrodial or synovial

11. Striated or skeletal

12. A motor neuron and the muscle fibers it supplies.

13. Insertion

14. A collection of tissues that work together to perform a specific function.

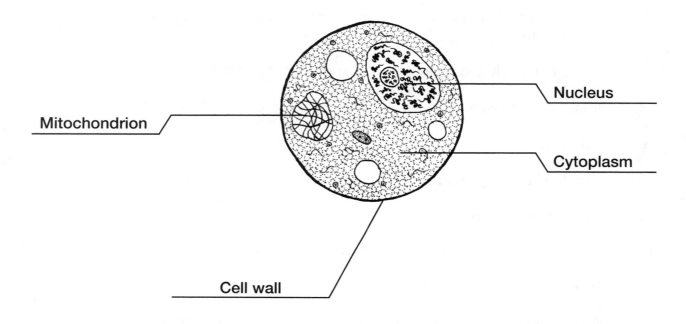

Mitochondrion

Nucleus

Cytoplasm

Cell wall

SOMATIC CELL

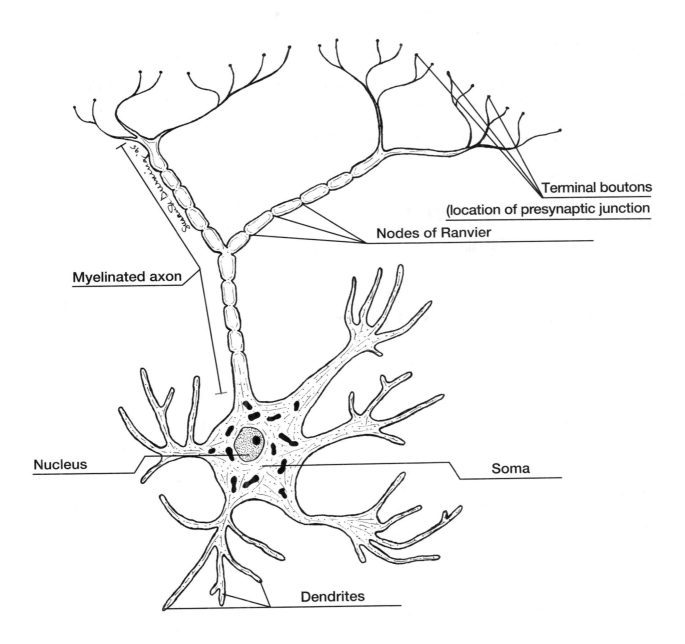

Terminal boutons
(location of presynaptic junction

Nodes of Ranvier

Myelinated axon

Nucleus

Soma

Dendrites

NEURON

1. Chemical and Biological

2. Volume; Boyle's Law.

3. a. Upper; b. Lower; c. Upper; d. Upper; e. Upper; f. Lower; g. Lower; h. Upper; i. Lower; j. upper

4. To provide compressed air for speech

5. The lungs and the respiratory passages

6. One inspiration and one expiration

7. 12 to 20 cycles/min.

8. The muscles of respiration

9. The diaphragm and the external intercostals

10. Relax

11. Cervical

12. Bucket handle movement

13. Forced expiration, such as blowing

14. Sternum

15. Spirometer

16. Thoracic

17. Tidal volume

18. Vital capacity

19. .16

20. Supplemental air; can be forcefully exhaled from resting expiratory level.

21. Diaphragmatic/abdominal; thoracic.

22.   Rapid, shallow cycles (tachypnea) gradually becoming longer and deeper (hyperpnea), followed by transient cessation of breathing (apnea). After this, the pattern repeats.

23.   Chronic obstructive pulmonary disease (COPD) is an irreversible condition in which the patient is unable to make optimal use of the oxygen in the air for respiration. Depending on the severity of the condition, the patient may be forced to speak in short utterances. Expiratory volume velocity may be insufficient to produce a normal voice. As the condition is irreversible, rehabilitation goals should be aimed at accommodation instead of recovery.

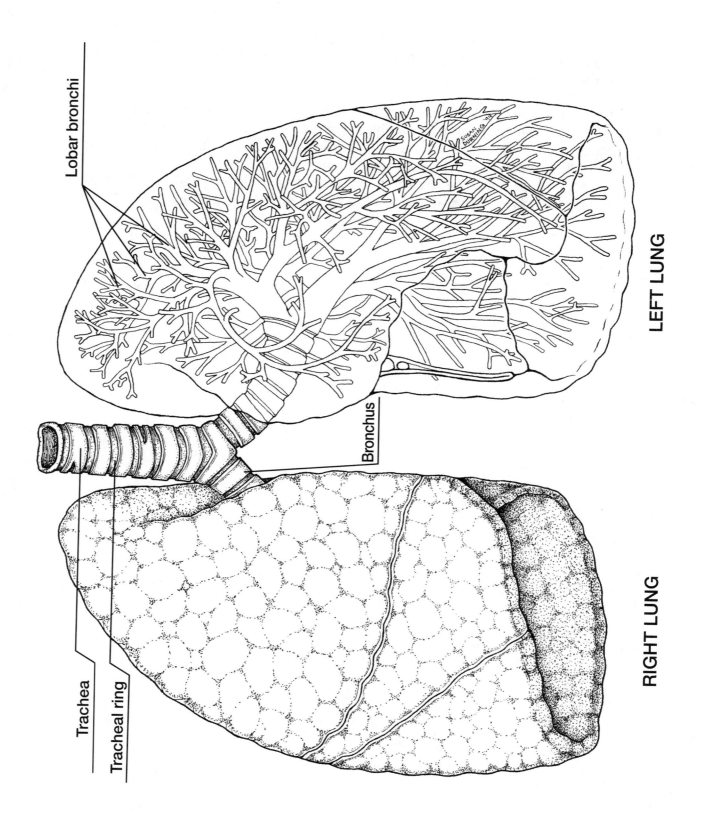

Lobar bronchi

LEFT LUNG

Bronchus

Trachea

Tracheal ring

RIGHT LUNG

6th cervical vertebra

1st rib

2nd rib

Sternum

External Intercostal muscles

Xiphoid process

Diaphragm

3rd lumbar vertebra

THORACIC SKELETON

1.   To protect the airway.

2.   Anterior

3.   To produce a phonatory source for speech.

4.   The complex tone produced when loosely approximated vocal folds emit pulses of pulmonary air.

5.   The number of times the glottis opens and closes in a given time.

6.   The amount of subglottic pressure

7.   The space between the vocal folds

8.   Skull

9.   The thyroid cartilage

10.   The cricoid cartilage

11.   Laminae (sing.: lamina)

12.   "Adam's apple"

13.   Cricoid cartilage

14.   The vocal processes of the arytenoid cartilages

15.   Abduction

16.   (d) Cricothyroid, thyroarytenoid, and vocalis muscles

17.   (a) Posterior cricoarytenoid muscles

18.   The muscular processes of the arytenoid cartilages

19.   Abducted

20.   Synovial

21.   Vocal ligament

22.   The intrinsic muscles are attached to laryngeal structures at both ends, whereas the extrinsic muscles are attached to laryngeal structures at one end and attached to other structures (i.e., the sternum) at the other end.

23.   The posterior cricoarytenoids

24.   To adjust the support, posture, and position of the larynx

25.   Subglottic pressure

26.   Approximately 210 Hz (Some authorities give 260 Hz)

27.   During phonation the glottis closes through combined myoelastic and aerodynamic forces. Myoelasticity is the tendency of the muscles to resist deformation. Aerodynamic forces result from the Bernoulli effect, or the tendency of the internal pressure of a liquid (such as air) to decrease as its velocity increases.

28.   The thyroarytenoid and vocalis muscles

29.   Superiorly

30.   Radiologists and speech-language pathologists observe cineradiographic studies of the upper airway during deglutition to note if any of the medium collects in the valleculae.

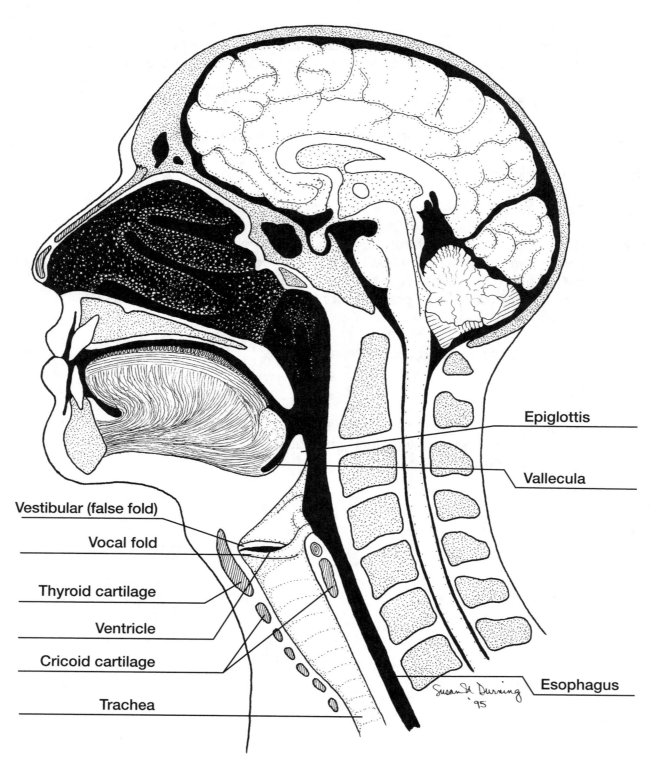

Epiglottis

Vallecula

Vestibular (false fold)

Vocal fold

Thyroid cartilage

Ventricle

Cricoid cartilage

Trachea

Esophagus

PHONATORY SYSTEM

392

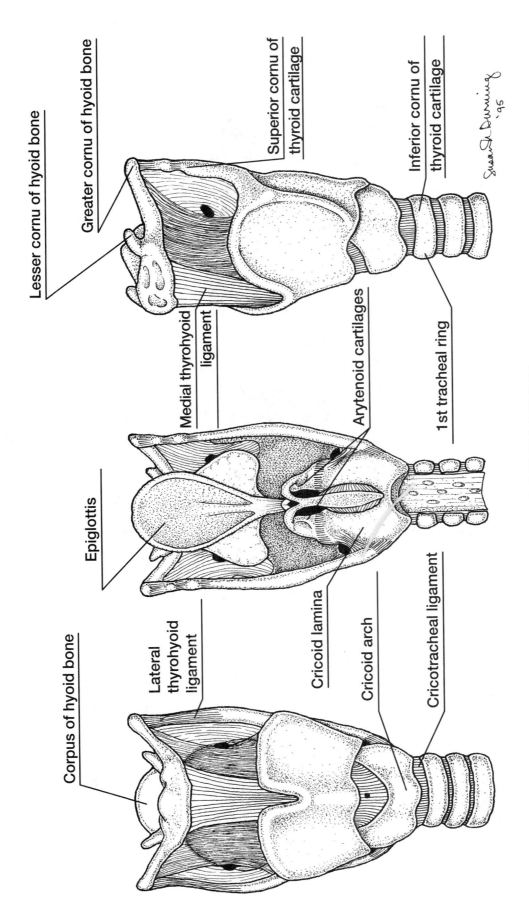

Lesser cornu of hyoid bone

Greater cornu of hyoid bone

Superior cornu of thyroid cartilage

Inferior cornu of thyroid cartilage

Medial thyrohyoid ligament

Arytenoid cartilages

1st tracheal ring

Epiglottis

Corpus of hyoid bone

Lateral thyrohyoid ligament

Cricoid lamina

Cricoid arch

Cricotracheal ligament

SKELETON OF THE LARYNX

393

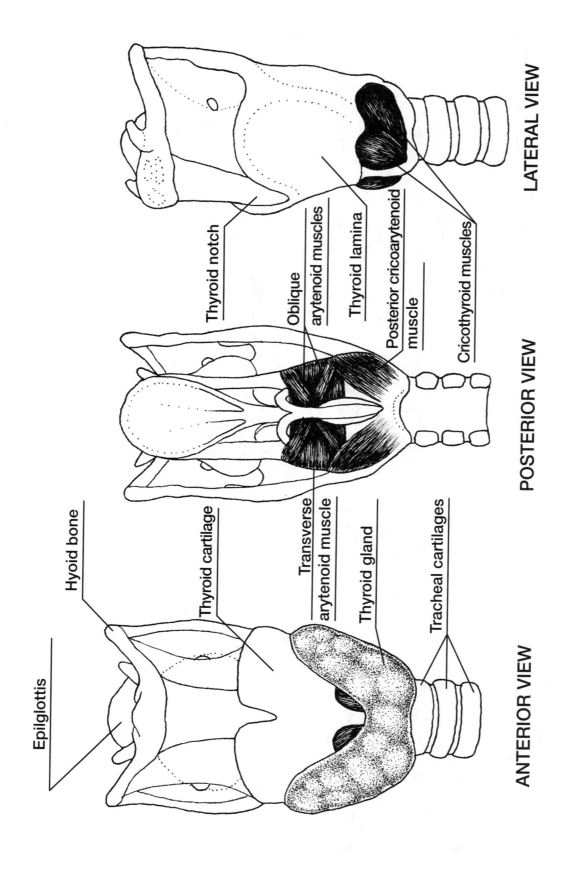

LATERAL VIEW

POSTERIOR VIEW

ANTERIOR VIEW

LARYNX

Thyroid notch

Oblique arytenoid muscles

Thyroid lamina

Posterior cricoarytenoid muscle

Cricothyroid muscles

Hyoid bone

Thyroid cartilage

Transverse arytenoid muscle

Thyroid gland

Tracheal cartilages

Epilglottis

394

1. Cranium

2. Frontal; temporal; sphenoid; parietal; occipital

3. Zygomatic

4. Mandible

5. Oral; nasal; pharyngeal

6. (Two) orbits, the nasal cavity, and the cranial cavity

7. The forehead (frons)

8. Palatoglossus muscles

9. Tongue; velum

10. "Cleft palate"

11. Orbicularis oris

12. Oral stage

13. Temporalis; masseter; and medial (internal) pterygoid muscles

14. Velum; tongue; mandible

15. Normally, with changes in dentition, the angle decreases as the individual reaches adulthood, then increases again as age advances and dentition is lost.

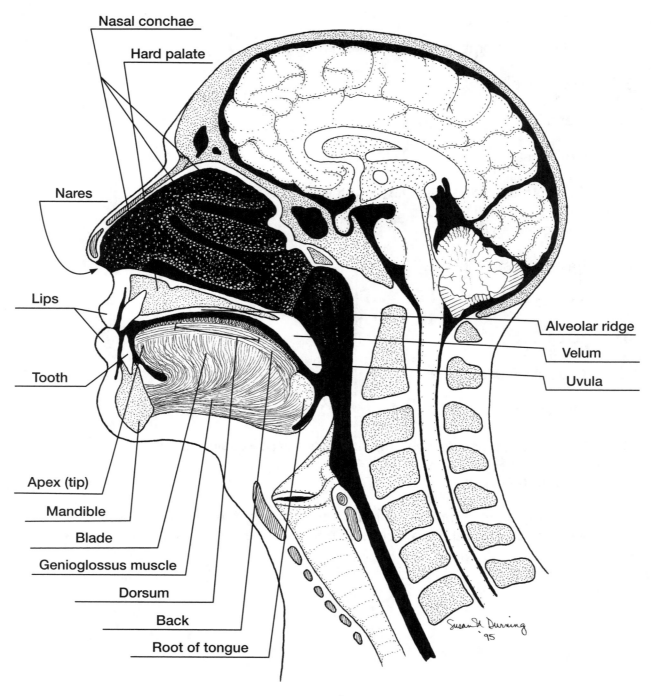

Nasal conchae

Hard palate

Nares

Lips

Tooth

Apex (tip)

Mandible

Blade

Genioglossus muscle

Dorsum

Back

Root of tongue

Alveolar ridge

Velum

Uvula

ARTICULATORY SYSTEM

396

Levator labii superioris muscle

Zygomaticus minor muscle

Zygomaticus major muscle

Orbicularis oris muscle

Levator anguli oris muscle

Risorius muscle

Depressor anguli oris muscle

Depressor labii inferioris muscle

MUSCLES OF FACIAL EXPRESSION

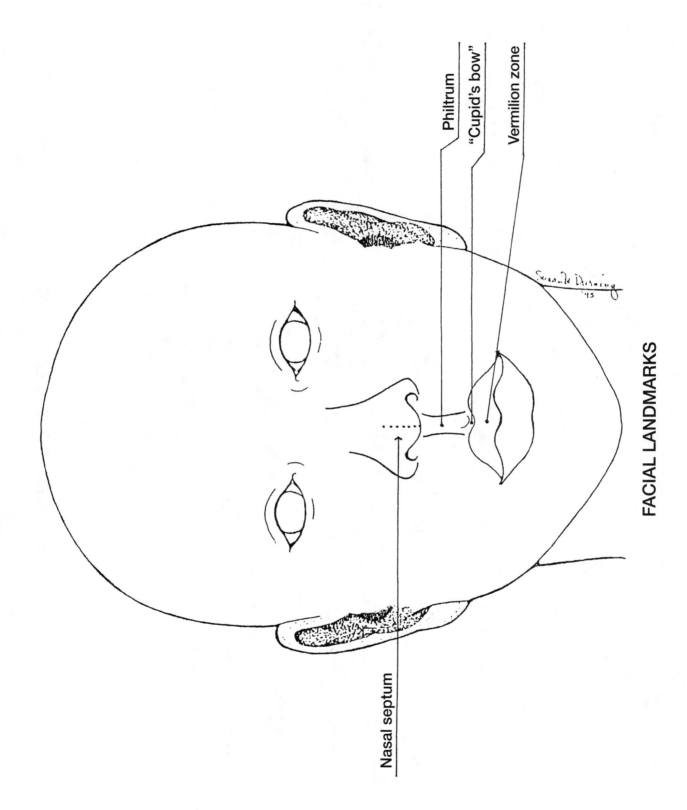

Philtrum

"Cupid's bow"

Vermilion zone

Nasal septum

FACIAL LANDMARKS

398

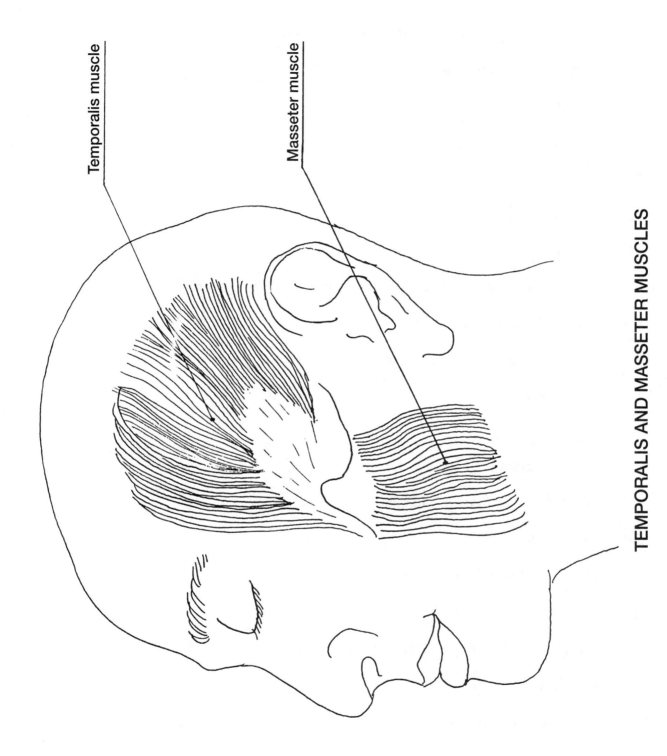

Temporalis muscle

Masseter muscle

TEMPORALIS AND MASSETER MUSCLES

399

1. Central nervous system and peripheral nervous system

2. The brain and the spinal cord

3. Afferent

4. Efferent

5. Frontal

6. 12

7. Peripheral

8. Spinal and cranial nerves and autonomic nervous system

9. Sympathetic nervous system

10. The association areas of the cerebral cortex

11. Synapses

12. Gyri

13. Lateral sulcus (fissure of Sylvius)

14. Central fissure (fissure of Rolando)

15. Sensory (tactile) reception

16. Pars triangularis of the left frontal lobe

17. Homonymous hemianopsia

18. Paralysis of the contralateral musculature

19. Brainstem

20. Hypoglossal nerve (XII).

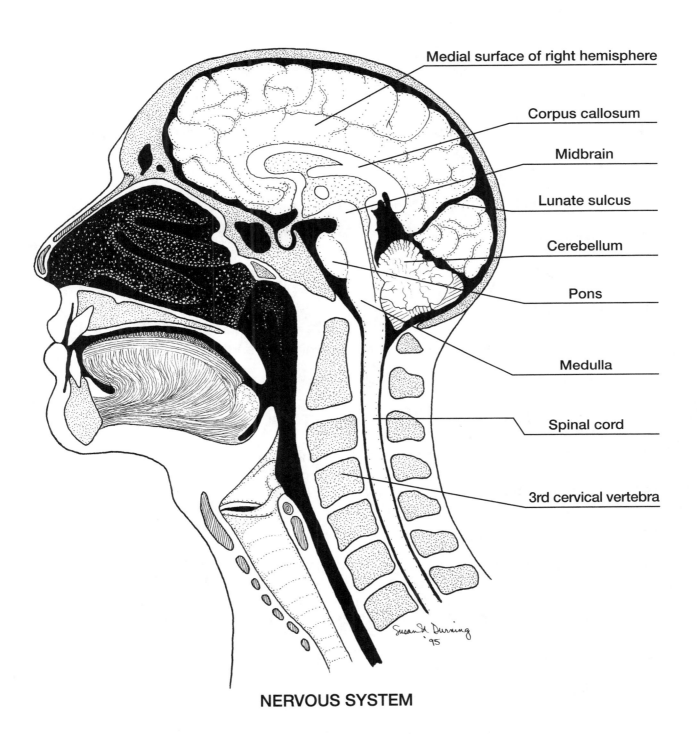

Medial surface of right hemisphere

Corpus callosum

Midbrain

Lunate sulcus

Cerebellum

Pons

Medulla

Spinal cord

3rd cervical vertebra

NERVOUS SYSTEM

1. Peripheral hearing mechanism

2. To direct acoustic energy to the external auditory meatus.

3. Cartilage

4. Match the acoustic impedance of the inner ear to that of the environment.

5. Malleus; incus; stapes

6. Eustachian (pharyngotympanic; auditory) tubes

7. Vestibular apparatus

8. Cochlea

9. Perilymph

10. Vestibulocochlear (acoustic) nerve or cranial nerve VIII

11. The pons

12. Superior olivary complex

13. Cerebral cortex of the dominant cerebral hemisphere

14. Temporal lobe

15. Cochlear nuclei

16. Acoustic neuroma

17. a) peripheral; b) peripheral; c) peripheral; d) central; e) central; f) peripheral;
    g) peripheral; h) peripheral; i) central; j) peripheral

18. Peripheral vestibular system

19. The malleus

20. The external ear: pinna: external auditory meatus and tympanic membrane; the
    middle ear: tympanic membrane, tympanic cavity, and eustachian tubes; and
    the inner ear: cochlea and vestibulocochlear nerve.

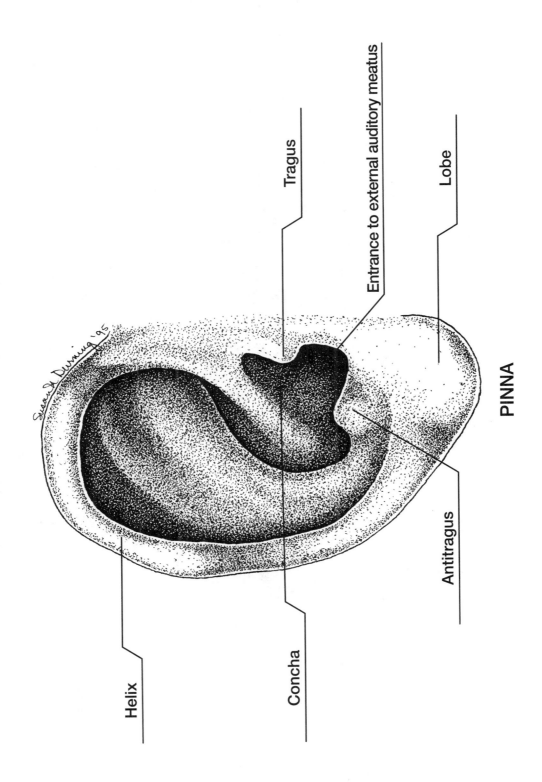

Tragus

Entrance to external auditory meatus

Lobe

Helix

Concha

Antitragus

PINNA

403

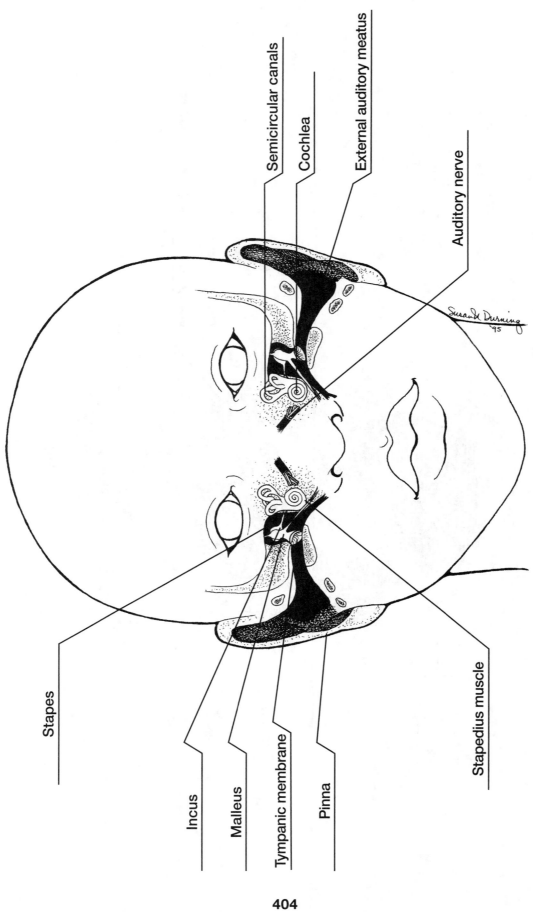

Semicircular canals

Cochlea

External auditory meatus

Auditory nerve

Stapes

Incus

Malleus

Tympanic membrane

Pinna

Stapedius muscle

CORONAL VIEW OF PERIPHERAL HEARING MECHANISM

404

INDEX